Clinical Cases in Paediatrics

Clinical Cases in Paediatrics

Nicholas P Mann MD MRCP DCH
Senior Registrar in Paediatrics
University Hospital
Queen's Medical Centre, Nottingham

Nicholas Rutter MD MRCP
Senior Lecturer in Child Health and
Honorary Consultant Paediatrician
The University of Nottingham

CHURCHILL LIVINGSTONE
EDINBURGH LONDON MELBOURNE AND NEW YORK 1986

CHURCHILL LIVINGSTONE
Medical Division of Longman Group UK Limited

Distributed in the United States of America by
Churchill Livingstone Inc., 1560 Broadway, New York,
N.Y. 10036, and by associated companies, branches
and representatives throughout the world.

© N P Mann and N Rutter 1986

All rights reserved. No part of this publication may be reproduced,
stored in a retrieval system, or transmitted, in any form or by any
means, electronic, mechanical, photocopying, recording and/or
otherwise, without the prior written permission of the publishers
(Churchill Livingstone, Robert Stevenson House,
1–3 Baxter's Place, Leith Walk, Edinburgh EH1 3AF).

First published 1986

ISBN 0 443 03660 8

British Library Cataloguing in Publication Data
Mann, Nicholas P.
　Clinical cases in paediatrics.
　1. Children—Diseases
　I. Title　　II. Rutter, Nicholas
　618.92　　RJ45

ISBN 0-443-03660-8

Printed in Great Britain at The Bath Press, Avon

Contents

Foreword		vii
Preface		viii

1 Clinical Genetics — 1
Down's Syndrome — 1
Klinefelter's Syndrome — 4

2 Neonatal Diseases — 6
Birth Asphyxia — 6
Prematurity — 8
Small for Dates Baby — 10
Respiratory Distress Syndrome — 12
Neonatal Jaundice — 14

3 Respiratory Diseases — 18
Common Cold — 18
Glue Ears — 18
Otitis Media — 20
Tonsillitis — 23
Croup — 23
Laryngomalacia — 25
Bronchiolitis — 26
Whooping Cough — 28
Asthma — 29
Tuberculosis — 31
Pneumonia — 34
Cystic Fibrosis — 36
Foreign Body Inhalation — 38

4 Cardiovascular Diseases — 41
Supraventricular Tachycardia — 41
Innocent Murmur — 42
Patent Ductus Arteriosus — 43
Coarctation of the Aorta — 45
Pulmonary Stenosis — 47
Ventricular Septal Defect — 48
Fallot's Tetralogy — 51

5 Gastroenterology — 53
Infectious Hepatitis — 53
Gastroenteritis — 54
Recurrent Abdominal Pain — 56
Herpes Stomatitis — 58
Hirschsprung's Disease — 59
Pyloric Stenosis — 60
Gastro-oesophageal Reflux — 64
Chronic Constipation — 65
Intussusception — 66
Coeliac Disease — 68
Acute Appendicitis — 69
Oesophageal Atresia — 71

6 Haematological Diseases — 74
Henoch–Schönlein Purpura — 74
Idiopathic Thrombocytopenic Purpura — 75
Haemophilia — 76
Iron Deficiency Anaemia — 77
Leukaemia — 79
Sickle Cell Disease — 80

7 Endocrine Diseases — 83
Short Stature — 83
Diabetes Mellitus — 86
Hypothyroidism — 88
Congenital Adrenal Hyperplasia — 91

8	**Renal Diseases**	**93**
	Urinary Tract Infection	93
	Vesicoureteric Reflux	94
	Bed Wetting	96
	Nephrotic Syndrome	97
	Chronic Renal Failure	99
9	**Infectious Diseases**	**102**
	Malaria	102
	Chickenpox	103
	Measles	104
	Congenital Rubella	105
	Acute Osteomyelitis	107
10	**Accidents and Trauma**	**109**
	Burns	109
	Non-accidental Injury	111
	Near-drowning	112
	Accidental Poisoning	114
	Head Injury	116
11	**Behavioural Problems**	**119**
	Temper Tantrums	119
	Overactive Child	120
	Teenage Suicide	121
	Anorexia Nervosa	122
12	**Surgery**	**124**
	Congenital Dislocation of the Hip	124
	Cleft Palate and Cleft Lip	125
	Irritable Hip	127
	Hypospadias	128
	Perthes' Disease	129
	Talipes	130
	Wilms' Tumour	131
13	**Skin Disorders**	**133**
	Nappy Rash	133
	Atopic Eczema	134
	Impetigo	136
14	**Neurological Disorders**	**137**
	Infantile Spasms	137
	Petit Mal Epilepsy	138
	Grand Mal Epilepsy	138
	Mental Handicap	140
	Hydrocephalus	142
	Duchenne Muscular Dystrophy	144
	Blindness	146
	Guillain–Barré Syndrome	147
	Meningitis	149
	Febrile Convulsion	151
	Cerebral Palsy	152
	Migraine	154
15	**Miscellaneous**	**156**
	Obesity	156
	Chronic Juvenile Arthritis	159
	Phenylketonuria	160
	Rickets	162
	Cot Death	164
	Food Intolerance	166
	Undescended Testis	167

Foreword

Teachers, often for their own comfort and convenience, elect to teach in their own particular way, likewise students learn in their own way. It is a happy school which 'gets its act together'. In Nottingham because of the pressure of the clinical services, paediatricians prepared statements and slide packages on common paediatric diseases as we understood them, to avoid repeatedly giving the same tutorial every eight weeks. These collections were published in *Essential Paediatrics* Hull D and Johnston D, Churchill Livingstone, 1981. We hoped that the clinical student would then be able to spend more time in A and E and OPD, and on the wards with the sick children and their families. Even so, the eight weeks allotted to paediatrics in the clinical course is but a brief time in which to acquire clinical experience. So to enliven and enrich the moments when students wait for children to be admitted, pathology results to become available, or surgical theatre to be prepared, Dr Nick Mann prepared a series of typical case reports of sick children: where they came from, how they fell ill, and what happened to them. They are not an alternative to seeing real children, but they do illustrate the way of things. The histories were accompanied by slide illustrations of the clinical features and pathological findings.

To make the material available for a wider audience, Dr Mann and Dr Rutter have modified the format so that it is suitable for publication. We all learn from individual examples and by trying to resolve particular problems, but these histories are not an alternative to a proper understanding of medical science or to wide practical experience. The aim of this book is rather to stimulate the former and complement the latter, and is written in a way that would be of help to any student of medicine, nursing, physiotherapy, etc, involved in caring for sick children.

David Hull
Professor of Child Health,
University of Nottingham

Preface

This book is a series of case reports covering the important illnesses which affect babies and children. Each report starts with the presenting symptoms and relevant features of the examination, and then describes the investigations which were performed. This is followed by a brief synopsis of the epidemiology, diagnosis and management of the illness. With a few minor modifications the case reports are those which we have collected and devised for our own Nottingham medical students to study during their two-month paediatric attachment. We hope that they will appeal to those who find it easier or more enjoyable to learn from examples of children with illnesses rather than from a conventional systematic textbook. Whilst they were written with medical students in mind, we hope they will be of interest to other professional groups who work with children—in particular, children's nurses, junior doctors, health visitors and therapists.

We are grateful to Geoff Lyth for his illustrations, Sue Emerson and Val Lowden for their typing and to the Nottingham paediatricians and paediatric surgeons (Professor D Hull, Professor A D Milner, Dr P Barbor, Dr D Johnston, Dr D Curnock, Dr E J Hiller, Dr D Mellor, Miss L Kapila and Miss M Mayell) for their support.

N P M
N R

1 Clinical genetics

Down's Syndrome

Denise, a child with Down's syndrome, has just had her fourth birthday. Her 24-year-old mother has recently divorced her husband, and has moved to be nearer the rest of her family. She is concerned about Denise's slow developmental progress and wishes to know whether any future children are likely to have Down's syndrome.

Denise is found to be a small, pleasant child with her height on the 3rd centile for her age and her head circumference just below the 3rd centile. Her face is round and she has upward-slanting eyes with marked epicanthic folds (Fig. 1.1). The nose is small with a flat bridge. The hands are broad but small with short fingers, especially the little fingers which are also in-curved (Fig. 1.2).

Examination of the palms reveals single transverse palmar creases (simian lines). During the neonatal period a wide gap between the first and second toes was easily recognized. Other common clinical features in these children are listed in Table 1.1.

Apparently Denise sat up at 9 months and was walking by 20 months. She can use a cup

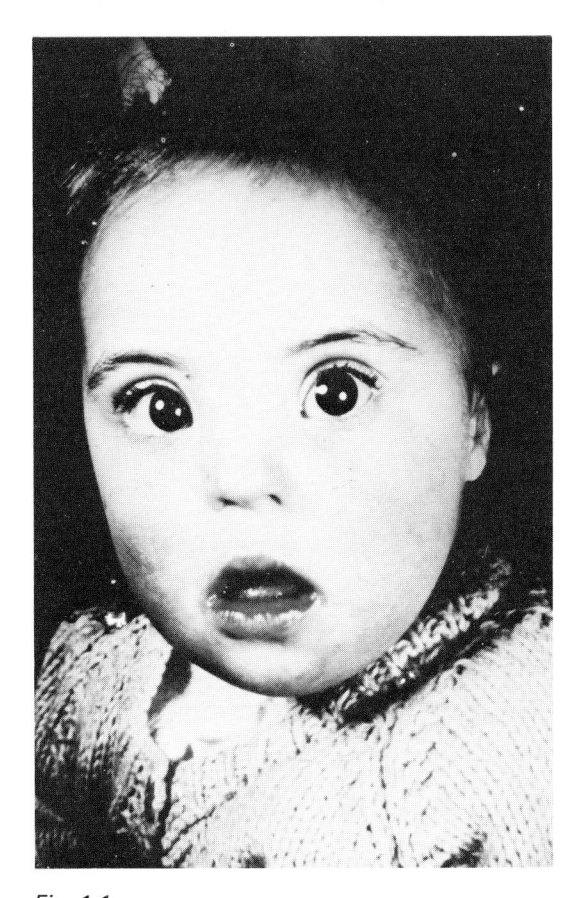

Fig. 1.1
Down's facies

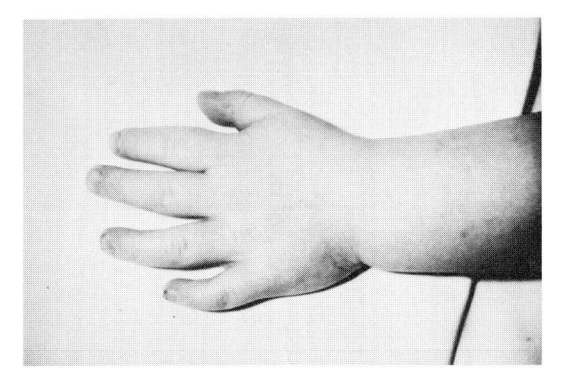

Fig. 1.2
Appearance of left hand in Down's syndrome

Table 1.1

Other clinical features of Down's syndrome

Flat occiput
Small mouth
Prominent fissured tongue
Simple ears
Irregular pigmentation of the iris
An increased incidence of congenital abnormalities (especially the heart and gastrointestinal tract)

and spoon to feed herself and says about five single words. She is partly potty trained, but still has 'accidents' during the day. Assessment reveals that she can build a tower of six cubes and will match colours, but will only scribble on paper rather than copy lines or a circle. Neurological examination reveals generalized hypotonia but no localized signs.

Comment

Denise is functioning at the level appropriate for a 2 year old, with particular delay in social and language skills. It appears that Denise is moderately retarded and that her mother has had unreal expectations of her future progress.

No chromosome analysis or genetic counselling had been previously offered. Down's syndrome is one of the commonest chromosome aberrations in the newborn, and karyotype examination revealed trisomy 21, which is associated with more than 90 per cent of cases (Fig. 1.3). This extra chromosome arises

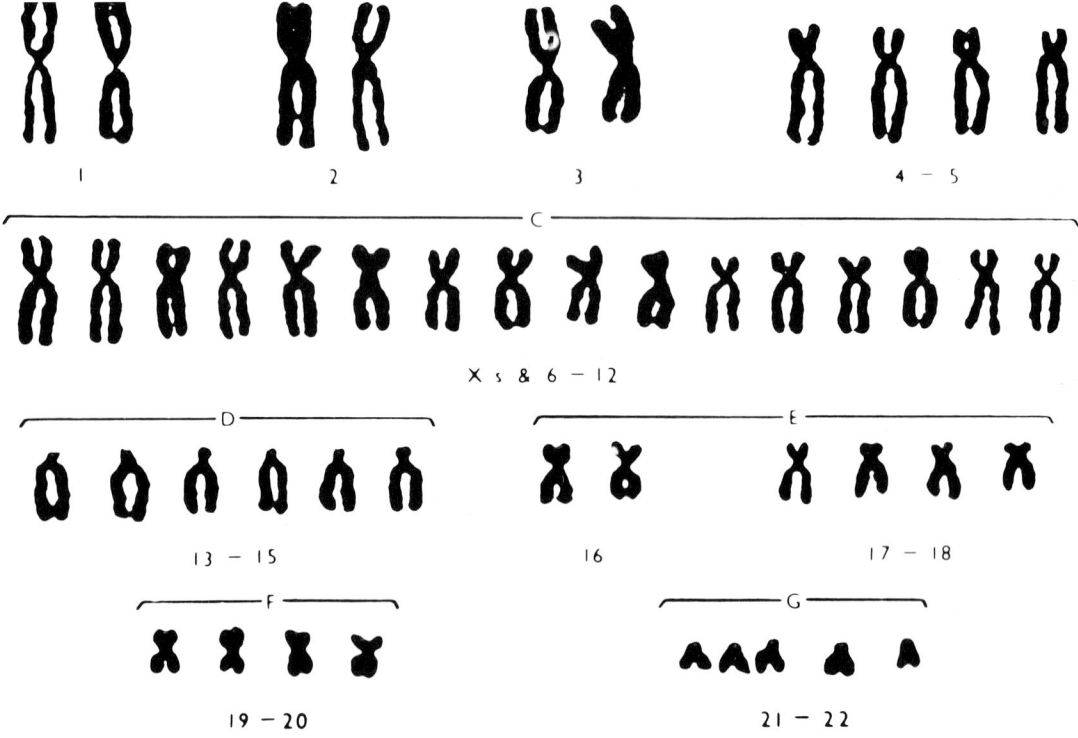

Fig. 1.3
Trisomy 21 karyotype

because of non-disjunction of chromosomes at meiosis, which produces some gametes with 24 chromosomes. Fertilization yields a zygote with 47 chromosomes, a risk closely related to maternal age (Fig. 1.4). Although the recurrence risk is low because of Denise's mother's age (<1 in 100), amniocentesis will be offered at 16 weeks' gestation with a future pregnancy. It is also recommended that all mothers over 35 years old be offered screening in this way.

Four per cent of cases of Down's syndrome are due to an unbalanced translocation, and a further 6 per cent due to mosaic formation; both of these have a far higher recurrence risk. For this reason, chromosome analysis and genetic counselling are mandatory in all cases of Down's syndrome. Other aspects of Denise's management are shown in Table 1.2.

Table 1.2

Management of child with Down's syndrome

Full information to parents
Genetic counselling
Team support by social workers, doctors and health visitors—if possible from community base
Access to toy library
Attendance allowance or invalidity pension
Special schooling or training facilities
Access to:
    Down's Children's Association
    Royal Society for the Mentally Handicapped (MENCAP)
Management of medical complications:
    congenital heart disease
    respiratory infections
    hypothyroidism

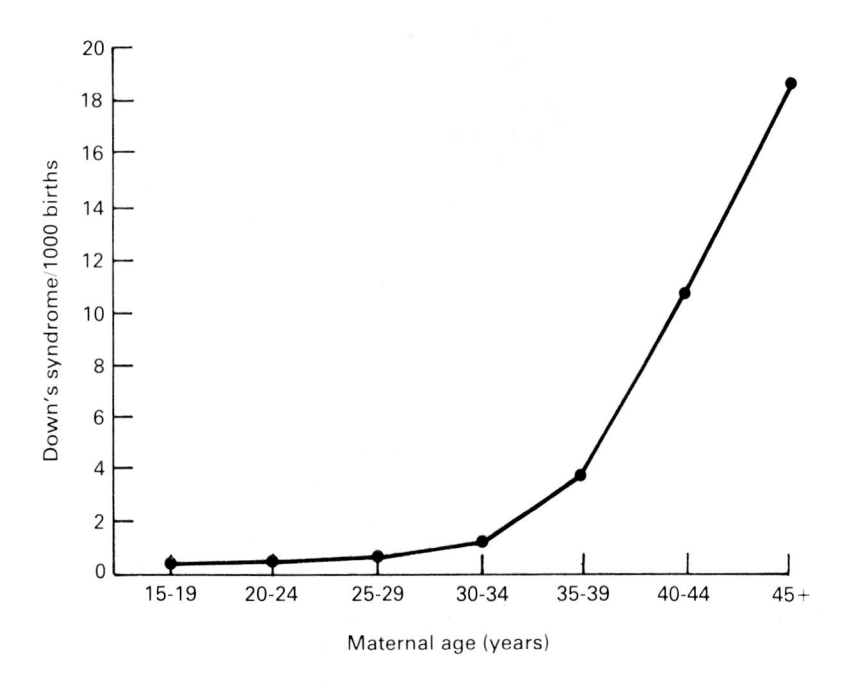

Fig. 1.4

Frequency of Down's syndrome in relation to maternal age

4 CLINICAL CASES IN PAEDIATRICS

Klinefelter's Syndrome

David, a 15 year old (Fig. 1.5), was referred to a general surgeon for advice about management of bilateral gynaecomastia, which had developed over the previous few months. His genitalia were noted to be very small on routine examination, and the surgeon felt that referral to the endocrine clinic was appropriate.

At this clinic David was noted to be a quiet, pleasant lad whose recent school performance had been rated as poor. Although his growth appeared normal with a height on the 50th centile for age, his arms were disproportionately long. There was no family history of similar problems and David's two older brothers were married with two children each. At examination pubic hair development was normal but both testes were of prepubertal size and the penis was small. A clinical diagnosis of Klinefelter's syndrome was tentatively made, and investigations showed the typical chromosomal appearance of this disorder as well as features of gonadal failure (Table 1.3).

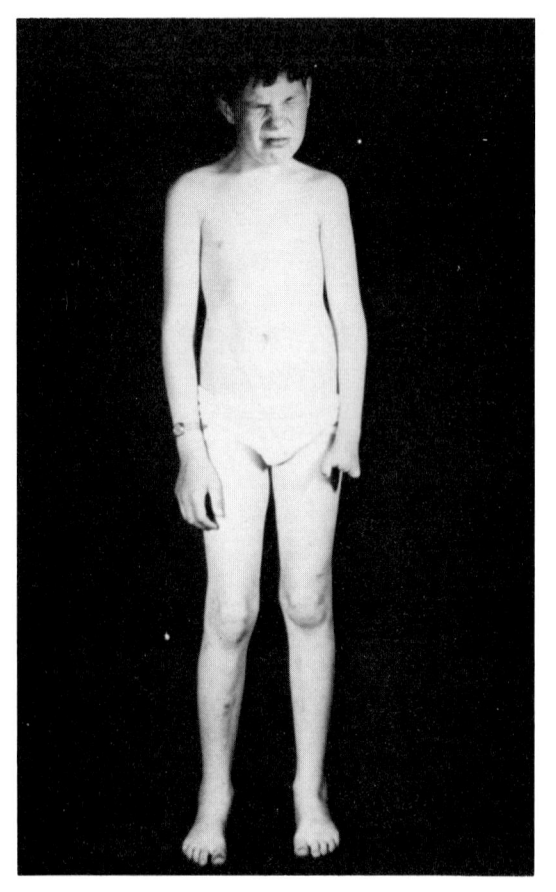

Table 1.3

Investigation in Klinefelter's syndrome

Karyotype:	47 chromosomes, with sex chromosomes XXY
Endocrine:	High plasma FSH and LH levels Low plasma testosterone

A detailed explanation was given to the family and genetic counselling arranged. A course of long-acting intramuscular testosterone injections was commenced.

Comment

Klinefelter's syndrome is the commonest specific chromosomal disorder and is the most frequent cause of male hypogonadism (all are infertile). The additional X chromosome arises through non-disjunction at meiosis in a similar way to Down's syndrome. Intellectual performance is frequently slightly reduced, with the mean IQ being 15–20 points below that of siblings.

Many cases are undetected even during adult life, but there are typical features which enable earlier diagnosis to be made (Table 1.4). Androgen deficiency leads to excessive height because of the failure of

Fig. 1.5
Klinefelter's syndrome

fusion of the epiphyses at puberty, and this is also responsible for obesity as an adult.

Table 1.4
Clinical features of Klinefelter's syndrome

Hypogonadism
   Small testes and penis, incomplete virilization, gynaecomastia, infertility
Growth:
   Children are often tall and slim
   Adults may be obese
Intelligence: IQ < 80 in 15%
Behavioural disturbance

Many cases are undetected, others are diagnosed at puberty or later

There is a high incidence of divorce, unemployment and alcoholism which are related to mental retardation, poor sexual performance and associated psychological disturbances.

Management involves discussion with the child at puberty and the use of replacement testosterone which will fuse the epiphyses and reduce gynaecomastia. There is now good evidence that androgen therapy will produce beneficial behavioural changes. Surgery for cosmetic purposes may be indicated if breast tissue is excessive in spite of such treatment. For the mother the risk of recurrence with future pregnancies is small, but most parents will have finished their families, since the diagnosis is made at puberty.

2 Neonatal diseases

Birth Asphyxia

Janet was born at term following a difficult delivery. Her mother, a 41-year-old primigravida, went into spontaneous labour which was slow to progress. Fetal distress developed after 16 hours, towards the end of the first stage of labour, so a Ventouse delivery was attempted. This failed, and a difficult mid-cavity forceps delivery ensued.

The paediatric houseman was presented with a pale, floppy, term baby who was not making any respiratory efforts. The baby was placed on a resuscitation trolley (Fig. 2.1) and the clock started. Auscultation revealed a heart rate of 20 per minute, and an Apgar score of 1, so the baby was intubated (Fig. 2.2). The endotracheal tube was connected to the oxygen supply which had a pressure-limiting valve set at 30 cm H_2O, and ventilation carried out at 20 breaths per minute by T-piece occlusion with a finger over the end of the tube.

The heart rate steadily increased to 120 per minute. However, it was five minutes before spontaneous respiration was established and the baby was extubated at eight minutes. Janet went to the postnatal ward with her mother where observations during the next few hours were satisfactory.

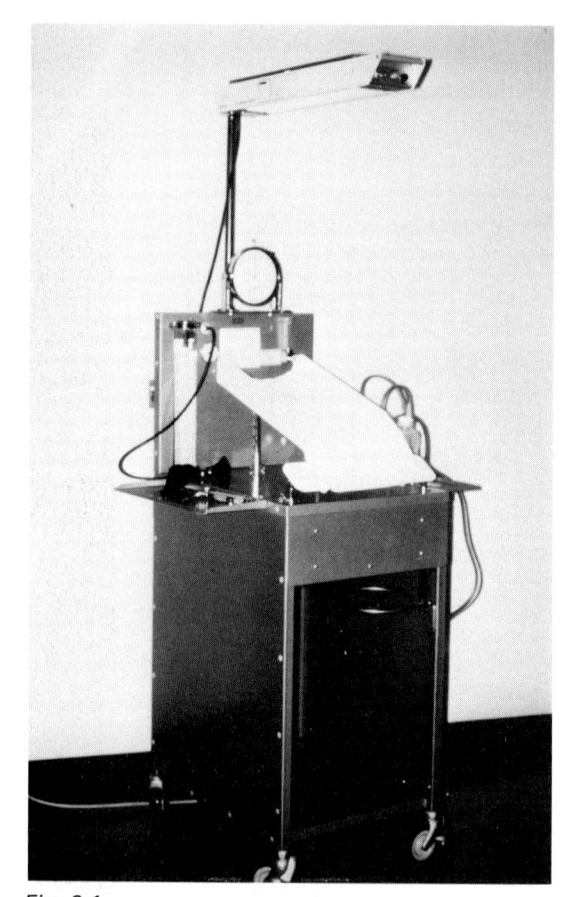

Fig. 2.1
Neonatal resuscitation trolley

Comment

Birth is the most dangerous time of life. The incidence and severity of perinatal asphyxia have decreased in recent years with improvements in maternal health and obstetric care. Under optimal conditions only 1–2 per cent of babies will require intubation and resuscitation. Numerous factors operate during labour and delivery to cause asphyxia.

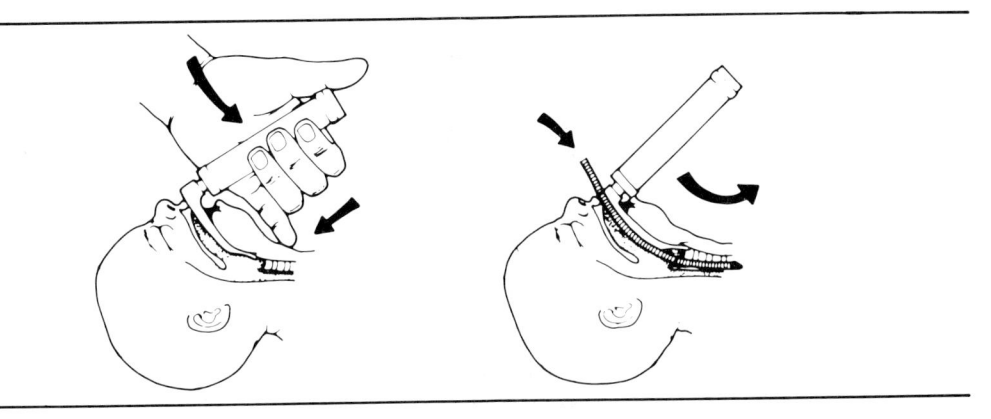

Fig. 2.2
Technique of intubation (*From Milner AD & Hull D (1984) Hospital Paediatrics. Churchill Livingstone, Edinburgh, by courtesy of the publishers*)

Janet was in terminal apnoea at birth and may not have survived without resuscitation. The Apgar score (Table 2.1) graded 0–10 is useful to assess the degree of asphyxia, but heart rate and spontaneous respiration are more useful than the other features. A heart rate below 60 per minute indicates severe asphyxia, whereas a rate over 100 per minute precludes this. Severe asphyxia is treated by intubation. Facemask resuscitation is commonly used for the treatment of less severe degrees of asphyxia.

Predisposing causes for asphyxia may be obvious, but birth asphyxia cannot always be predicted (Fig. 2.3). The occasional death following home delivery is a tragedy. Perinatal asphyxia accounts for up to 20 per cent of the perinatal mortality, as many stillbirths are the result of intrauterine asphyxia. It is a sad fact that many maternity units still operate with staff who are insufficiently trained in neonatal intubation and resuscitation techniques.

Sometimes the sequelae of severe asphyxia are an irritable or convulsing neonate who is hypertonic and dislikes being handled. Alternatively, cerebral asphyxia may lead to a floppy, lethargic infant. These neurological signs often disappear within a few days, and the most reliable estimate of prognosis in an individual baby follows a neurological exami-

Table 2.1
Apgar score

	0	1	2
Colour	Blue, pale	Trunk pink, limbs blue	All pink
Pulse	Absent	<100	>100
Reflex response	None	Grimace	Cry
Tone	Limp	Some flexion	Active movement
Respiration	Absent	Slow, irregular	Strong

8 CLINICAL CASES IN PAEDIATRICS

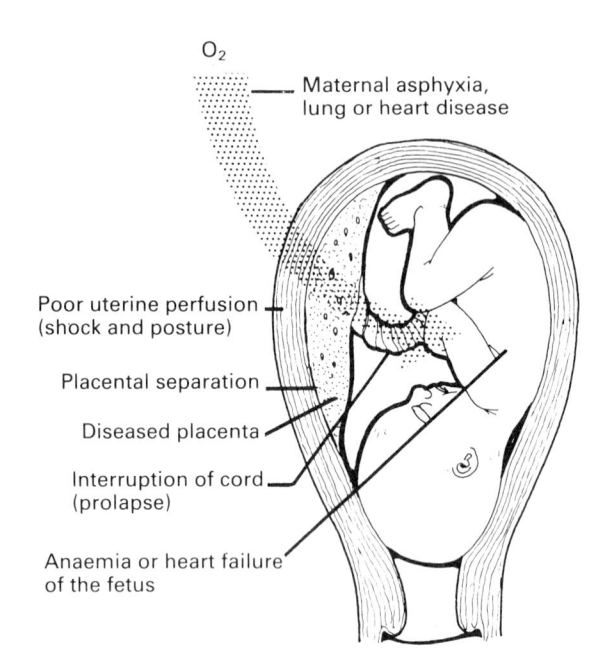

Fig. 2.3
Predisposing factors to birth asphyxia

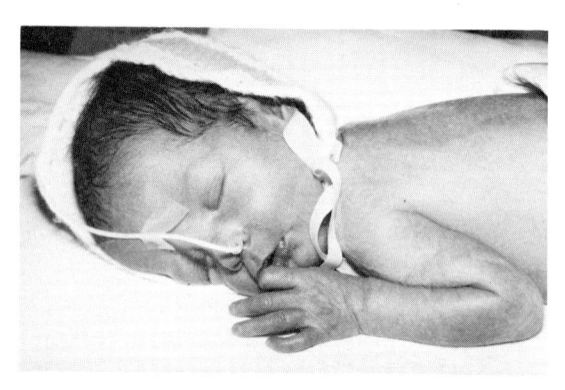

Fig. 2.4
Typical preterm baby

nation at 2–3 weeks. If grossly abnormal, there is a high incidence of cerebral palsy but fortunately in many cases the signs have disappeared and an optimistic outlook can be given.

Prematurity

Peter was born at 32 weeks' gestation with a birth weight of 1.42 kg. His mother, a primigravida, had been admitted in premature labour and her cervix was 5 cm dilated on arrival in hospital. An epidural anaesthetic was given and three hours later she delivered the baby with the assistance of forceps. He was in good condition at birth and was taken to the neonatal unit.

A gestational assessment of maturity agreed with his mother's dates. Peter was nursed naked in an incubator on an apnoea mattress (set to alarm after ten seconds of apnoea) and attached to an ECG monitor. A nasogastric tube was inserted and continuous milk feeds were commenced at 2–3 ml per hour with donor breast milk at four hours when his condition was found to be stable (Fig. 2.4).

All went well until the fifth day when a low grade fever, vomiting and two cyanotic episodes were noted. An infection screen was carried out (Table 2.2), feeds were stopped and intravenous gentamicin and flucloxacillin were commenced. The situation settled rapidly, the infection screen was subsequently found to be negative and the antibiotics were discontinued.

Peter started growing by 2 weeks and had no major problems during his stay. He had jaundice of prematurity which was treated

Table 2.2

Screening a preterm infant for an infection

The following investigations are necessary:
  Blood culture
  Urine culture
  Lumbar puncture
  Chest x-ray
  Blood count

with phototherapy on days four to seven. Fortunately he was well enough to be clothed by 10 days so he could come out of his incubator for short periods for a cuddle and chat with his mother and father. He graduated to a cot at 4 weeks and was discharged home with a weight of 2.2 kg at 8 weeks of age.

Comment

The mean birth weight in the United Kingdom is 3.30 kg, and 6 per cent of infants are born weighing less than 2.50 kg; these are classified as *low birth weight*, irrespective of gestation. Clearly this may arise if the baby is born early (preterm infant) or if he is underweight in relation to age (small for dates) (Table 2.3). The possible complications that arise in these two groups are very different (Table 2.4).

Table 2.3

Low birth weight (below 2.50 kg)

Preterm (born before 37 weeks' gestation)	65%
Small for dates (weight below 10th percentile for gestation)	35%

Survival of very low birth weight babies weighing less than 1.50 kg (1 per cent of live births) provides a major challenge to those involved in the care of the newborn, as survival decreases dramatically below this weight. Survival has steadily improved during the last 20 years, and major handicap such as blindness, deafness and cerebral palsy are now less common. Better obstetric care, prompt treatment of birth asphyxia, conservation of body temperature and adequate nutrition play a central role in this improvement. Techniques for respiratory support developed since the mid-1960s have produced further reductions in morbidity and mortality, so that there is now a 50 per cent chance of survival in an infant weighing 1.00 kg at birth.

The importance of bonding between mother and infant has been emphasized recently. When visiting to a neonatal unit is restricted and the baby is shut away in a Perspex box, it is easy to see how failure to bond together arises. Rituals such as the routine wearing of masks and gowns by staff are more likely to cause barriers to communication than to bacteria. Open visiting, 'hotel' facilities for parents and photographs of the baby, as well as encouragement and involvement with routine nursing and encouraging other children

Table 2.4

Complications in low birth weight infants

Preterm	Small for dates
Respiratory distress syndrome	Birth asphyxia
Apnoea	Meconium aspiration
Jaundice	Hypoglycaemia
Impaired temperature control	Polycythaemia
Persistent ductus arteriosus	Congenital malformations
Infection	Congenital infections
Intraventricular haemorrhage	
Haemorrhagic disease	
Functional bowel obstruction	

in the family to visit (Fig. 2.5) appear to help during this crucial period of development.

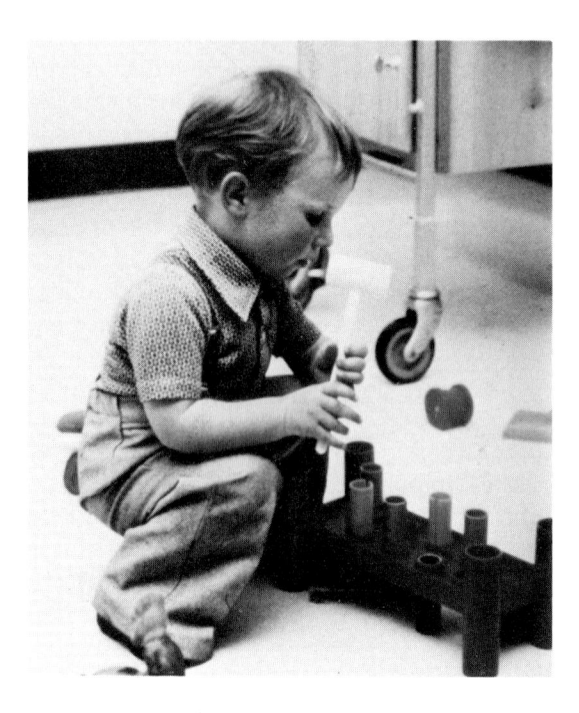

Fig. 2.5
Play facilities on neonatal unit

Small for Dates Baby

Brett was born at 38 weeks' gestation weighing 1.85 kg (well below the 10th centile for age at this gestation). The pregnancy had been complicated by pre-eclampsia, so repeated ultrasound scans were carried out to assess fetal head growth. These showed growth in the biparietal diameter but at a slower rate than expected (Fig. 2.6). An elective caesarean section was carried out at 38 weeks because of a failed induction of labour, which was undertaken because of worsening placental function tests.

The baby was in good condition at birth and was transferred to the neonatal unit for observation. There was no evidence of chromosomal abnormality or congenital infection. Height, weight and head circumference were all below the 10th centiles for age (Fig. 2.7). Feeding was commenced shortly after birth and capillary glucose levels were monitored from heel pricks. Brett was mainly bottle fed, but required some nasogastric feeding for a week. He was discharged home after two weeks weighing 1.98 kg. A health visitor with a special interest in the newborn was able to visit the home on a regular basis to give help and advice to the parents.

Comment

There are a wide variety of causes for small size, but in practice most are unknown (Table 2.5). The infant may be thin but with a normal head size, reflecting adequate brain growth *in utero*, as the brain is preferentially protected. With more severe growth failure, especially if chronic, head circumference will be low.

Energy stores such as glycogen may be insufficient for the stresses of prolonged labour, so fetal distress and birth asphyxia may be severe. Problems may arise before the onset of labour and the incidence of stillbirth is high.

Follow-up studies show that a significant proportion remain small throughout life. By the age of 4 years, about a third of such children have a weight and height below the 3rd centile, but growth of an individual child is difficult to predict. Clearly there are concerns about brain growth and function in the longer term. There appears to be a high frequency of school problems associated with speech delay and minimal brain dysfunction even when intelligence is normal. Again these are impossible to predict in an individual.

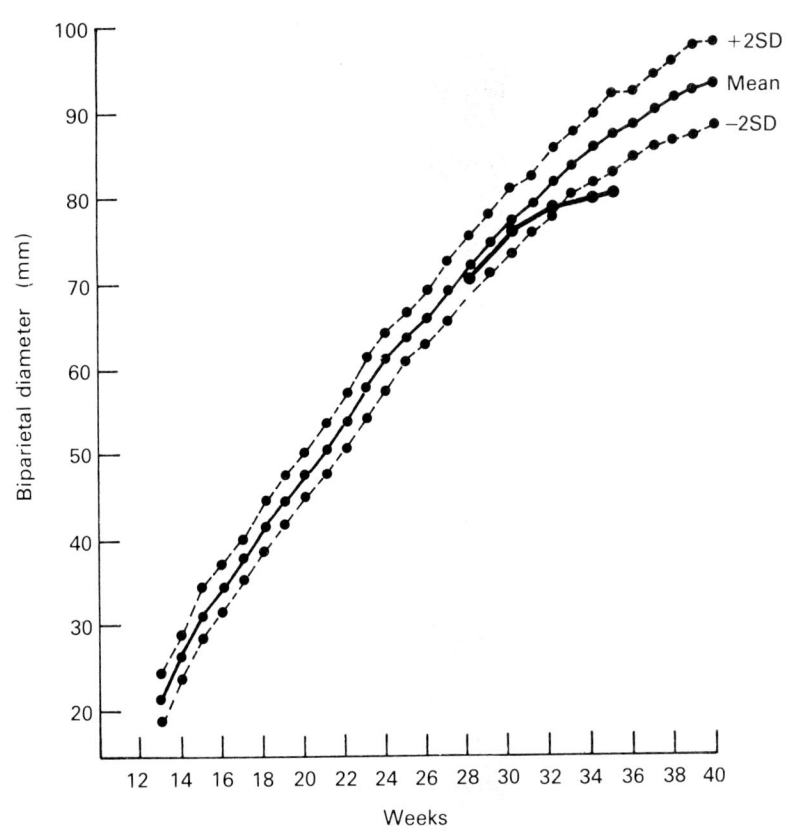

Fig. 2.6
Biparietal head diameter measurements in growth-retarded fetus

Long-term follow-up seems sensible to pick up such problems at an early stage when help from speech therapists or educational psychologists can be recruited. Fortunately, only a small proportion of small for dates infants are due to intrauterine infection or chromosomal

Table 2.5
Aetiology of the small for dates infant

Maternal factors	Infant factors
Multiple pregnancy Low socioeconomic class Smoking Alcohol Malnutrition Pre-eclampsia	Congenital infection (e.g. rubella) Chromosomal abnormalities Genetic factors (short parents, particularly the mother)

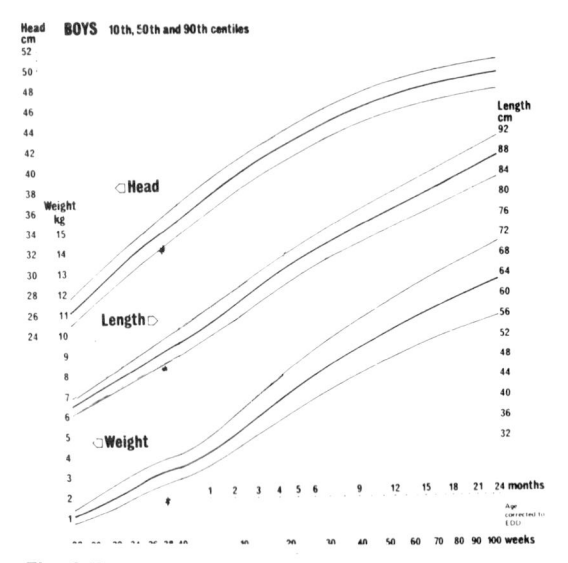

Fig. 2.7
Typical growth chart of small for dates infant

abnormality where cerebral function is likely to be grossly abnormal.

Respiratory Distress Syndrome

Elizabeth was born at 28 weeks' gestation and weighed 0.91 kg. She was asphyxiated at birth and required ventilation with oxygen via an endotracheal tube for four minutes before breathing spontaneously. On transfer to an incubator her respiratory rate was 80 per minute and there was sternal and intercostal recession. In view of this, an umbilical arterial catheter was sited in the aorta to obtain regular samples for blood gas analysis and to monitor blood pressure. The catheter tip was too high (Fig. 2.8) so the catheter was withdrawn to a position just above the diaphragm.

At the age of 3 hours, Elizabeth became apnoeic and was commenced on mechanical ventilation (Fig. 2.9). The chest x-ray showed a ground glass appearance of the lung fields with bilateral air bronchograms, more pronounced on the right than the left side. It was felt she had idiopathic respiratory distress syndrome (IRDS, hyaline membrane disease). Intravenous benzylpenicillin was given to cover the possibility of group B streptococcal pneumonia.

A slow improvement took place during the next few hours of ventilation but suddenly the baby collapsed with peripheral shutdown and a poor volume pulse. A chest x-ray was taken which showed a large tension pneumothorax (Fig. 2.10). The response to insertion of a chest drain was dramatic.

Elizabeth spent four weeks on the ventilator and nine weeks in hospital. Cranial ultrasound examinations did not show any evidence of intraventricular haemorrhage. She appeared to be making excellent progress by the time of discharge, and the parents were given a guardedly good prognosis.

Comment

One-third of admissions and half of the deaths in newborn intensive care units are due to respiratory problems. IRDS associated with surfactant deficiency is the commonest of these, and is common in infants below 32 weeks' gestation. Typical clinical manifestations develop within hours of birth (Table 2.6) and enable classification into mild, moderate or severe disease. Pneumonia caused by group B streptococcal disease is

Table 2.6

Idiopathic respiratory distress syndrome

A disease of preterm infants, characterized by the early onset of:
    Tachypnoea
    Expiratory grunting
    Subcostal, intercostal and sternal recession
    Widespread lung crackles
    Central cyanosis

NEONATAL DISEASES 13

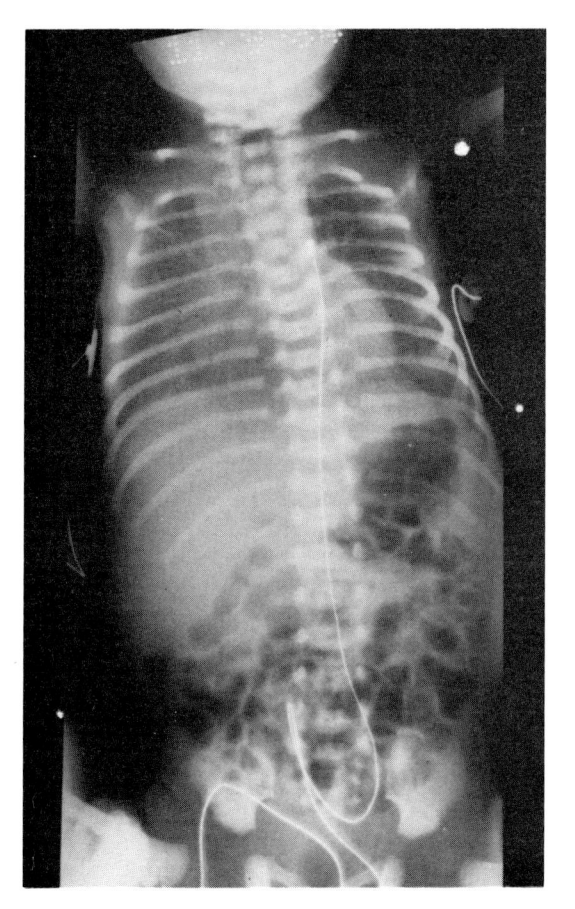

Fig. 2.8
X-ray showing umbilical arterial catheter

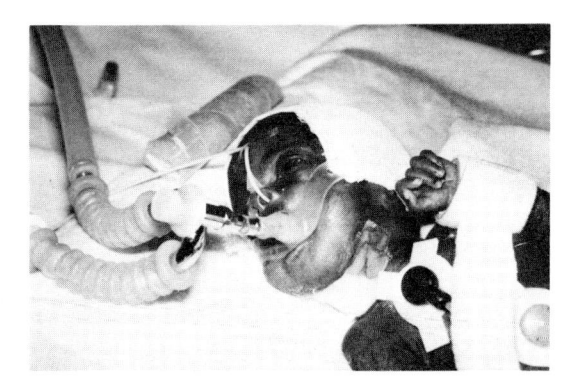

Fig. 2.9
Neonate receiving mechanical ventilation

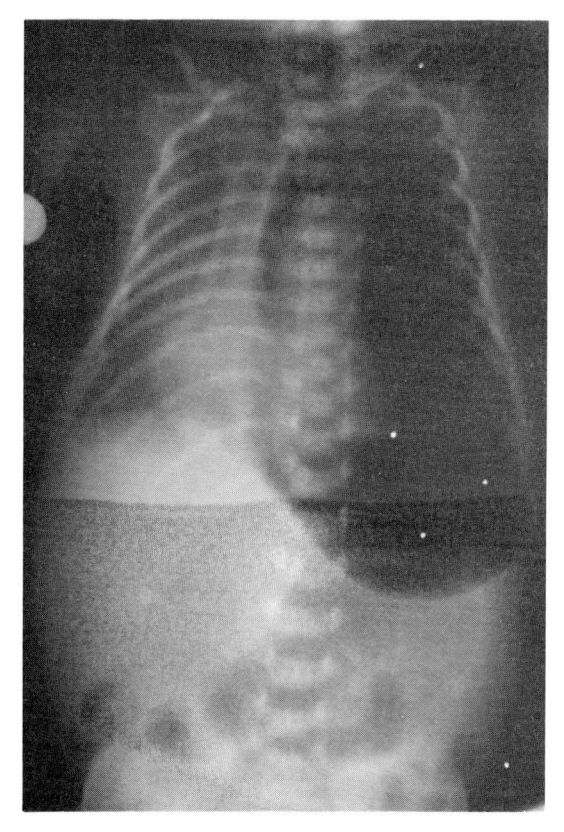

Fig. 2.10
Tension pneumothorax

impossible to distinguish from IRDS, so penicillin is given to all moderate or severe cases.

A tension pneumothorax is a sudden, life-threatening complication which can be diagnosed by fibreoptic light examination. The affected side of the chest glows like a lantern. In this way the pneumothorax can be drained immediately without the delay involved in x-ray procedures. Treatment of IRDS involves the use of oxygen by headbox (Figs. 2.11 and 2.12), continuous positive airway pressure (CPAP) or ventilation (Fig. 2.13). Oxygen therapy is monitored by measurement of the inspired oxygen concentration in conjunction

Fig. 2.11

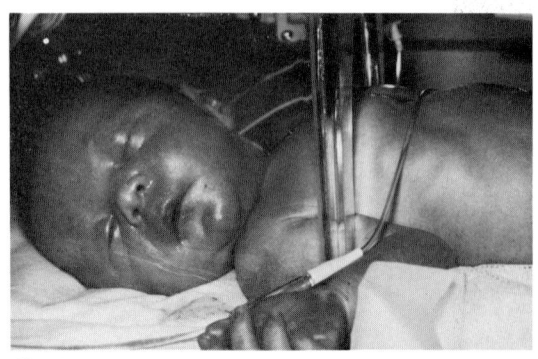

Neonate receiving oxygen via a headbox

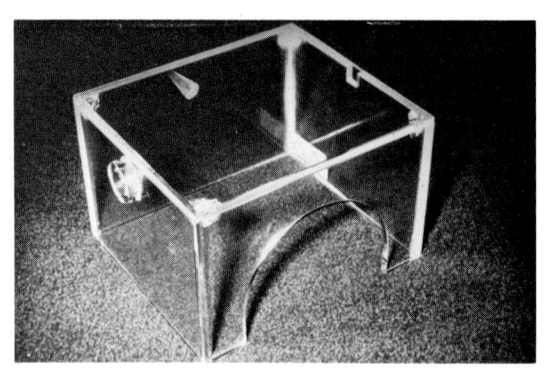

Fig. 2.12

Headbox for oxygen therapy

with blood oxygen tension measurement. Arterial blood samples for direct Pao_2 measurement can be taken from an arterial line and analysed in a blood gas machine. Additionally, transcutaneous capillary oxygen tension can now readily measured on a continuous basis. High arterial oxygen tensions predispose to the development of permanent eye damage in the form of retrolental fibroplasia.

Dramatic improvements in neonatal intensive care with wider availability have improved the outlook for IRDS, and most survivors should have normal intellectual development and be left without handicap.

Neonatal Jaundice

Raina, who was born by a normal delivery at term weighing 3.30 kg, was noted by a nursery nurse at 3 days to be jaundiced and rather sleepy. Her parents were of Kenyan Asian origin. The paediatric houseman was called to the ward to find a well but rather sleepy baby who had apparently been slow to feed. It was difficult to assess the degree of jaundice, but the gums and conjunctivae looked moderately yellow. The rest of the examination was normal. Raina's mother was upset to think that her baby needed medical attention.

A capillary blood sample was taken from a heel prick, and to the doctor's surprise the bilirubin level was found to be 335 µmol/l. In view of the high bilirubin level, further investigations were performed. These showed that nearly all the bilirubin was unconjugated and the blood group of both mother and baby was O positive. Other investigations were normal. It was felt that Raina had physiological jaundice and phototherapy was commenced (Fig. 2.14) after an explanation to the mother. Fluid intake was boosted to prevent dehydration as the baby had had insufficient intake of milk during the previous day. The bilirubin level remained static for 12 hours and then declined. Phototherapy was stopped on the fifth day and the baby was discharged home on the eighth day.

Comment

Jaundice in the newborn is extremely common in the first week of life. Jaundice becomes visible with a bilirubin over 85 µmol/l in Caucasian babies, but is more difficult to recognize in Asian or Negro infants. With experience it is possible to judge if the level exceeds about 170 µmol/l, when laboratory measurement is needed.

It is important to decide on the aetiology

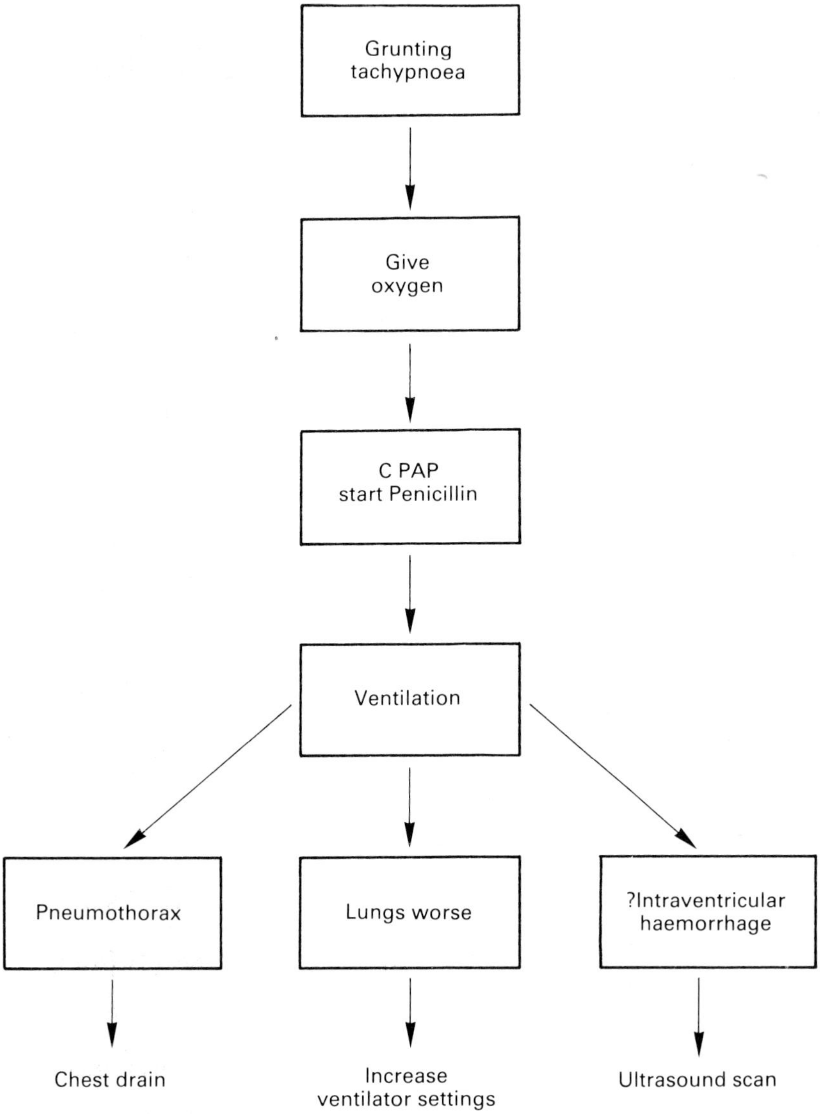

Fig. 2.13
Management of respiratory distress syndrome

of jaundice, which will vary with age (Table 2.7). Jaundice in the first 24 hours of life must be assumed to be due to haemolysis until proved otherwise, and needs urgent investigation and treatment. After 24 hours the most common type is physiological (a diagnosis of exclusion), and this is frequently exacerbated by bruising from obstetric trauma or cephalhaematoma (Fig. 2.15).

Management of jaundice in the newborn

16 CLINICAL CASES IN PAEDIATRICS

Fig. 2.14
Phototherapy unit (*From Milner AD & Hull D (1984)* Hospital Paediatrics. *Churchill Livingstone, Edinburgh, by courtesy of the publishers*)

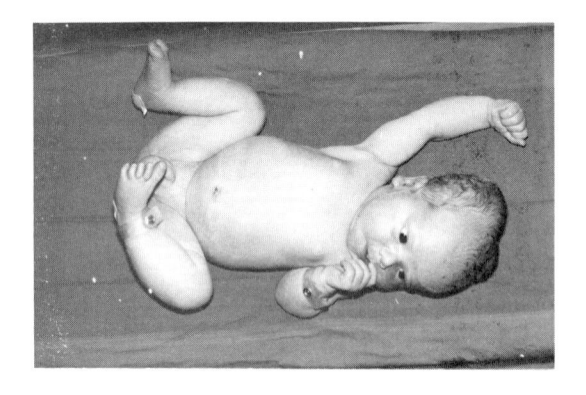

Fig. 2.15
Bilateral cephalhaematomas

involves treatment of the underlying cause (e.g. infection), and prevention of kernicterus (Fig. 2.16), which leads to death or brain damage. This is the deposition of unconjugated bilirubin (fat soluble) in the brain, and may occur in untreated or inadequately treated rhesus disease, particularly if the infant is preterm and ill. Phototherapy is used to treat jaundice by degradation of unconjugated bilirubin in the skin with exposure to light in the blue–green visible spectrum (wavelength 450 nm) produced from fluorescent tubes. The indications for its use are shown, as well as those for exchange transfu-

Table 2.7

Aetiology of neonatal jaundice

1 day	2–10 days	More than 10 days
Haemolysis (rhesus disease) ABO incompatibility Glucose-6-phosphate dehydrogenase deficiency	Physiological Prematurity Polycythaemia Bruising Infections (especially urinary tract)	Breast milk jaundice Hypothyroidism Hepatitis } conjugated Biliary atresia } jaundice

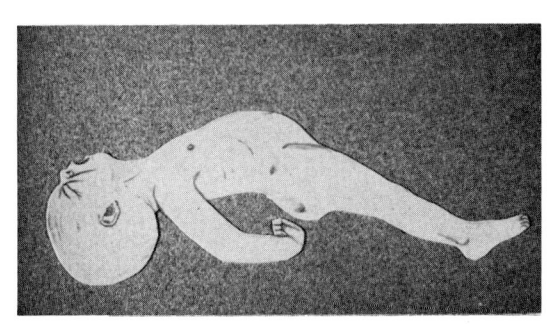

Fig. 2.16
Opisthotonus in kernicterus

Table 2.8

Treatment of jaundice in the newborn

Term infant:
  Phototherapy if bilirubin exceeds 320 μmol/l
  Exchange transfusion if bilirubin exceeds 375 μmol/l

Preterm infant below 30 weeks' gestation:
  Phototherapy if bilirubin exceeds 100 μmol/l
  Exchange transfusion if bilirubin exceeds 175 μmol/l

sion, in Table 2.8. The risk of kernicterus has probably been overstated in recent years and these bilirubin levels are higher than previously recommended.

The prognosis for physiological jaundice is excellent. Fortunately, the majority of cases do not require investigation or treatment.

3 Respiratory diseases

Common Cold

Teresa, a 2 year old, had a snotty nose for several days with coughing at night. Apart from a poor appetite she was reasonably well. Her parents were concerned and brought her along to the surgery because this was the eighth such infection she had had in the past year and they wanted to know how to prevent further episodes. On further questioning, it became clear that Teresa was never free of snuffles. On examination there was no evidence of tonsillitis, otitis media or lower respiratory tract involvement, but she was noted to sneeze several times and to rub her eyes.

Comment

Upper respiratory infections of all kinds in children show a seasonal variation, being most common in winter and spring. Children often have up to six or eight infections annually, with some episodes accompanied by constitutional symptoms such as fever and malaise. Symptoms of a cold may also precede infections such as croup, bronchiolitis and measles, so parents must contact their doctor if new symptoms develop. Occasionally a nasal discharge in a toddler may be unilateral, blood stained and foul smelling. A foreign body in the nose should then be considered. In children under 1 year of age, constitutional symptoms are common during a cold, so particular care will be needed to exclude other infections such as pneumonia or meningitis.

Colds are caused by a variety of viruses which give rise to inflammation of the nasal mucosa with excessive production of secretions. Teresa probably has an allergic inflammation of the nasal mucosa, perennial rhinitis, as well as her cold. This combination of allergy and superimposed infection is very common in children. The older child with perennial rhinitis can be treated with a steroid nasal spray. There is no satisfactory way of reducing the incidence of colds, and further investigations are not needed.

Treatment of a cold is frequently unnecessary. Aspirin or paracetamol can be used for constitutional symptoms. There is no evidence that antibiotics or antihistamines have any beneficial effects. If the nose is becoming obstructed, especially in infants who are obligate nose breathers and therefore have difficulty in feeding, a decongestant such as xylometazoline 0.05% (Otrivine) can be used for a few days to shrink the mucosa and reduce nasal secretions. Parents should be made aware that symptoms from a cold may persist for up to two weeks so that repeated visits to the doctor are avoided.

Glue Ears

John was referred for hearing assessment at the age of 6 years by his school medical officer. He was born at term following a normal pregnancy and delivery with a birth weight of 3.3 kg. The routine hearing test carried out by the distraction method at 8 months had been normal. John's speech had been delayed so that he was only able to say a few words at 3 years of age, but his mother said he acquired an extensive vocabulary shortly afterwards. Both mother and teacher commented that John had a short attention span. At a screening 'sweep test' of hearing John failed to hear any of the four pure tone sounds presented to him.

The ENT surgeon found retracted eardrums which were opaque so that the ossicles could not be visualized. Pure tone audiometry showed typical features of conductive deafness, with a hearing loss of 40 decibels (dB), confirming the surgeon's diagnosis of glue ears (secretory otitis media).

Since a six-week course of antibiotics and decongestants was ineffective, grommets were placed in the eardrum to drain the middle ear and an adenoidectomy was carried out.

Comment

Hearing loss is traditionally divided into conductive (36 per 1000 children) and perceptive hearing loss (1 per 1000 children). In children, glue ears make up the vast majority of conductive losses and recessively inherited deafness about half of the perceptive losses. Some children are at high risk of deafness, and will need a low index of suspicion for a formal hearing assessment by a trained audiometry technician (Table 3.1). Such testing is especially difficult in the younger handicapped child, but equipment such as sound level meters enable the intensity of various sound stimuli to be measured accurately.

The distraction hearing screening tests already described are routinely undertaken by health visitors at the age of 8 months so that severe deafness can be treated before language development is delayed (Fig. 3.1). The 'sweep' screening test soon after school entry should enable hearing loss secondary to glue ears to be recognized in order to avoid educational and behavioural difficulties at school. (There are few symptoms from glue ears.)

Table 3.1
Factors carrying an increased risk of deafness

Cerebral palsy
Cleft palate
Very low birth weight (below 1.50 kg)
Family history of deafness
Following meningitis

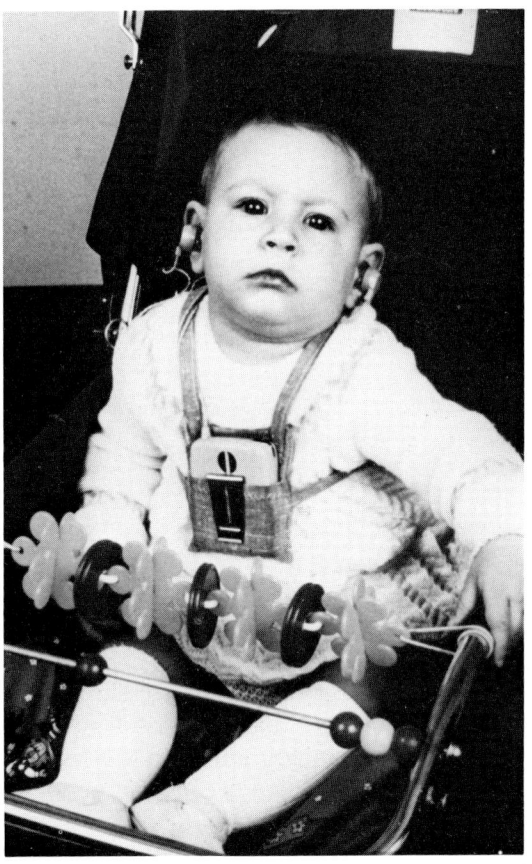

Fig. 3.1
Infant with hearing aids

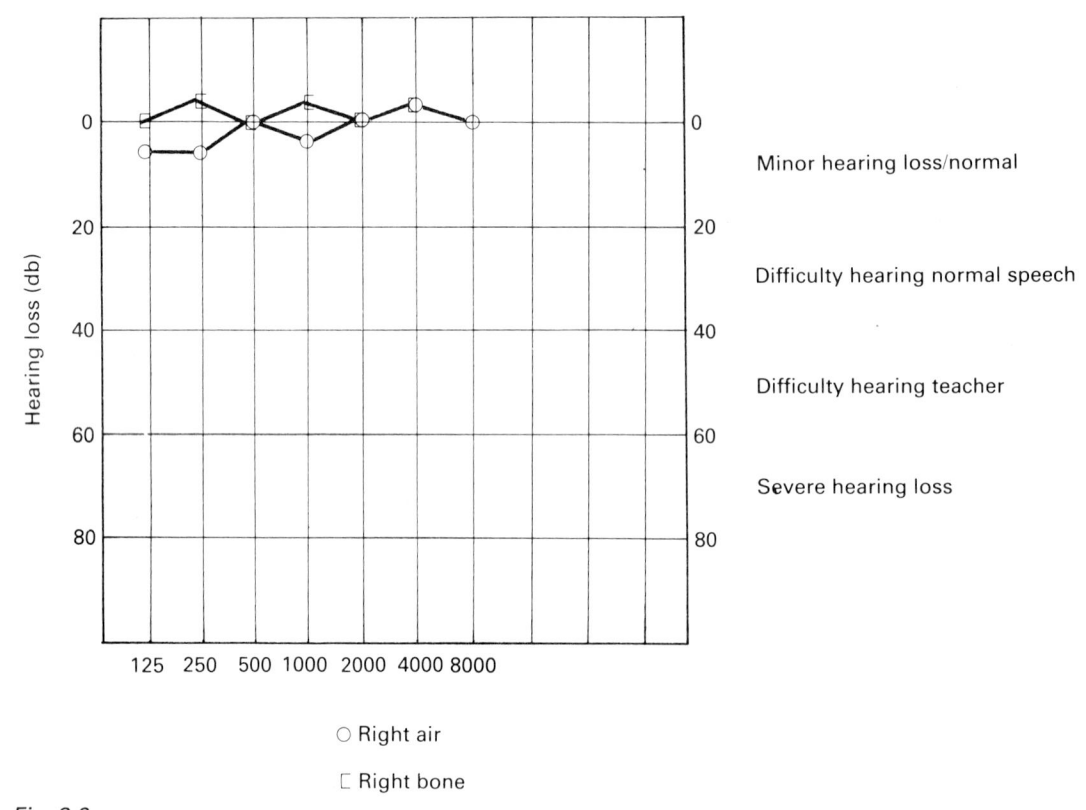

Fig. 3.2

Normal audiogram, showing scale for measuring deafness in decibels (dB)

Pure tone audiometry measures bone and air conduction separately in both ears, a technique that can be applied to a child with a mental age of more than 3 years. Figure 3.2 shows a normal audiogram, with the hearing loss in decibels that can occur from minor to severe deafness. The scale is a logarithmic function. The child with conductive loss due to glue ears shows a relatively larger loss of air than with bone conduction (Fig. 3.3).

Treatment of glue ears is still controversial as no method produces entirely satisfactory results. John's hearing loss improved dramatically in the first few weeks postoperatively but a 30 dB loss was still present a year later. He was sat in the front row at school to enable him to hear the teacher more clearly. The condition tends to resolve during childhood and is rarely seen after 12 years of age.

Otitis Media

Amanda, aged 18 months, was seen with a 12-hour history of a fever of 39°C and vomiting. During the last four months she had had five episodes of otitis media and her mother thought these symptoms were similar to those on previous occasions. On examination (Figs. 3.4 and 3.5), her eardrums were red and congested with an absent light reflex. A seven-day course of amoxycillin was commenced,

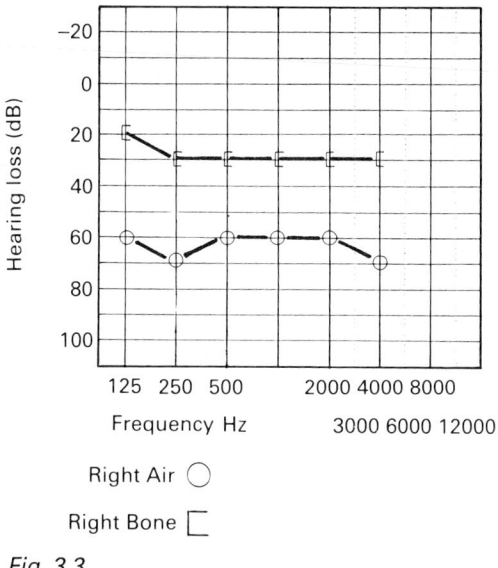

Fig. 3.3
Audiogram in conductive deafness

with advice on the use of paracetamol to control pain and fever. Amanda was reviewed two weeks later. Prophylactic antibiotics were started using once daily co-trimoxazole because of the frequency of infection. The GP suggested using this treatment for the rest of the winter.

Comment

Otitis media is a common complication of a cold or infectious disease in young children, and more than half of children will have had one more infection by the age of 2 years. It appears that infection enters the middle ear by spreading up the eustachian tube whose function is impaired during a cold. The symptoms produced by otitis media will be dependent on age, as a child under 4 years is unable to localize pain to his ear. Ear pulling by infants and young children is notoriously unreliable as a feature of ear infection. *Examination of all ill children must include inspection of the eardrums with an auroscope.*

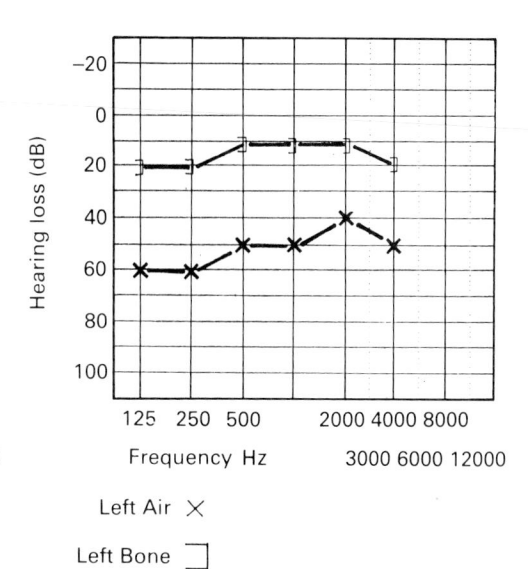

Two-thirds of cases are caused by bacterial infection and one-third by mycoplasma or viral infection. The common bacterial pathogens are shown in Table 3.2. Suitable antibiotics are amoxycillin, co-trimoxazole and erythromycin.

With repeated episodes of otitis media,

Table 3.2

Bacteria which cause acute otitis media

Pneumococcus
Streptococcus (β-haemolytic)
Haemophilus influenzae
Staphylococcus aureus
Bacteroides Sp.

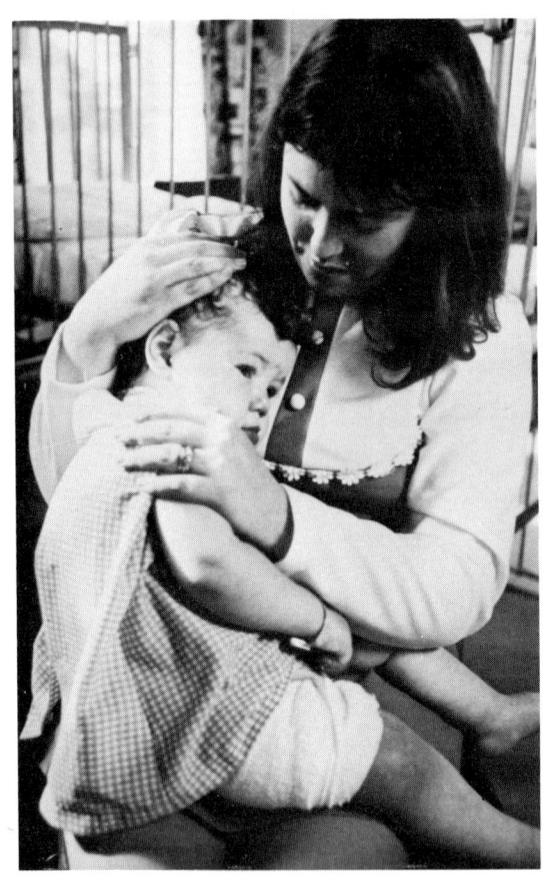

Fig. 3.4
Holding a child for examination of ears

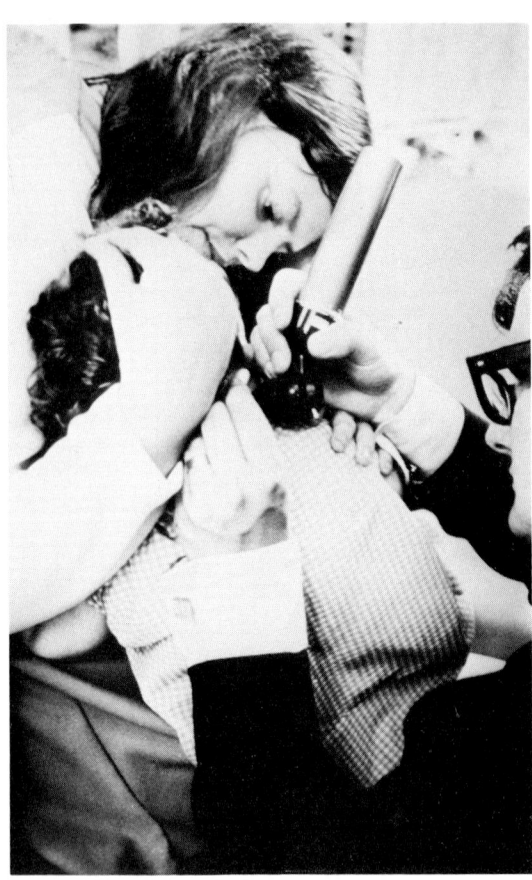

Fig. 3.5
Technique for examination of ears

hearing impairment may last several months and the risk of developing glue ear increases. There is no evidence to suggest that tonsillectomy or adenoidectomy reduces the incidence of repeated infection, but beneficial effects have been demonstrated from prophylactic antibiotics. Acute otitis media used to be treated by myringotomy in order to enable drainage of pus from the middle ear. It is a painful unpleasant procedure that is now rarely used. In untreated middle ear infections, pressure necrosis of part of the eardrum will produce spontaneous drainage of pus and a discharging ear.

The possibility of glue ear must be considered when deafness or other symptoms are present several weeks after treatment. However, the prognosis for acute otitis media is excellent and complications are rare. They occur when infection spreads locally to the mastoid air cells (mastoiditis) or intracranially (meningitis, cerebral abscess). Chronic suppurative middle ear disease used to occur before antibiotic treatment was available.

Tonsillitis

Marie, a 3 year old, developed a febrile illness of sudden onset associated with vomiting and abdominal pain. The family doctor who was asked to see Marie found a temperature of 39.8°C and tender enlarged cervical lymph nodes. She also noted that the pharynx was inflamed and that the tonsils were covered with small purulent spots. There was no evidence of otitis media when the ears were inspected with an auriscope.

She gave a five-day course of penicillin and suggested using aspirin or paracetamol to control the fever and discomfort. The symptoms settled over the next two days and Marie was able to return to her nursery a few days later.

Comment

Pharyngitis/tonsillitis is one of the commonest infections in children. The young child may not accurately localize the pain, and abdominal pain is relatively common as with any febrile illness. The majority of cases have a viral aetiology, but by far the commonest bacterial pathogen is the β-haemolytic streptococcus. The appearance of the throat does not help distinguish between these infective agents. Routine throat swabs are not cost effective and serve very little useful purpose. A white slough covering the tonsils may suggest glandular fever, and ulceration of the fauces an infection due to Coxsackie A virus. Complications of tonsillitis occasionally arise (Table 3.3).

About 150 000 tonsillectomies a year are carried out in the UK costing the National Health Service millions of pounds. There is little scientific basis for carrying out many of these operations and occasional deaths do occur. Different doctors examining a group of children are unable to decide consistently which child should be recommended for tonsillectomy. There are, however, a few indications where there can be major benefits following removal of the tonsils (Table 3.4). The evidence that any arbitrary number of sore throats in a year is reduced following tonsillectomy is extremely thin! Further research is needed in this area to decide whether the operation should be relegated to the category of an obsolete ritual (like routine circumcision, or incision of tongue tie).

Croup

Joanne, aged 22 months, was brought up to the accident and emergency department at 2:00 a.m. by anxious parents who had noted a harsh barking cough for several hours associated with noisy breathing. She had had a cold for two days but had been reasonably well until the breathing difficulty. The clinical

Table 3.3
Complications of tonsillitis

1–7 days	Over 7 days
Peritonsillar abscess (quinsy) Retropharyngeal abscess Cervical abscess Otitis media Scarlet fever	Rheumatic fever Acute glomerulonephritis

Table 3.4
Indications for tonsillectomy

Upper respiratory tract obstruction leading to sleep apnoea
Suspected malignancy
Peritonsillar abscess (quinsy)

findings were those of moderate stridor during inspiration, with supraclavicular and substernal recession, and a 'barking' cough. There were no signs of cyanosis and the axillary temperature was 37.4°C.

In view of the degree of stridor, hospital admission was arranged for close observation of respiratory status. The child's condition remained stable overnight and the stridor disappeared the next day, but returned the following night, albeit in a milder form.

Comment

The history is typical of laryngotracheobronchitis (croup), which is usually seen in children from 6 months to 3 years of age and commonly appears after the onset of an upper respiratory infection. Obstruction to the airway is due to swelling and inflammation of the subglottic region of the larynx. The obstruction is worse on inspiration (Fig. 3.6) and therefore results in inspiratory stridor. Several viruses can cause croup (Table 3.5).

Table 3.5
Viruses which cause croup

Parainfluenza virus (the commonest)
Respiratory syncytial virus
Influenza virus
Measles virus

The management of the child with stridor depends on the diagnosis (Fig. 3.7). In practice, this generally means distinguishing croup from acute epiglottitis, although a foreign body obstructing the larynx must always be considered when the obstruction is of sudden onset. Lateral x-rays of the neck are occasionally helpful in distinguishing croup from epiglottitis but it must be emphasized that an examination of the mouth with a spatula in severe stridor is likely to precipitate respiratory arrest.

The treatment of the child with croup is minimal intervention, and involves keeping the child settled, preferably with the mother living in on the ward. No benefits have been found from the use of antibiotics, steroids or humidified air, and routine oxygen will mask

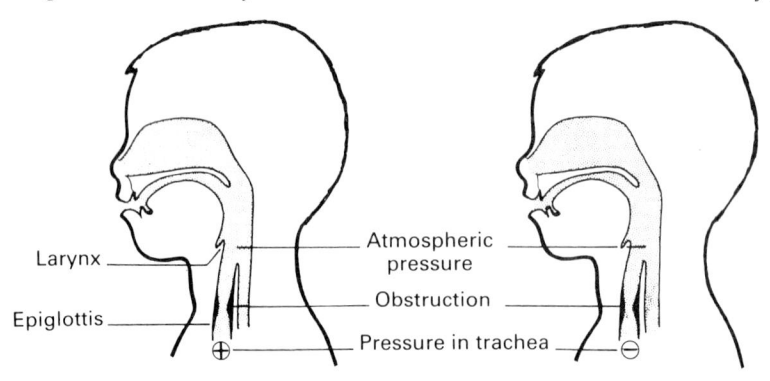

Fig. 3.6
Mechanism of stridor

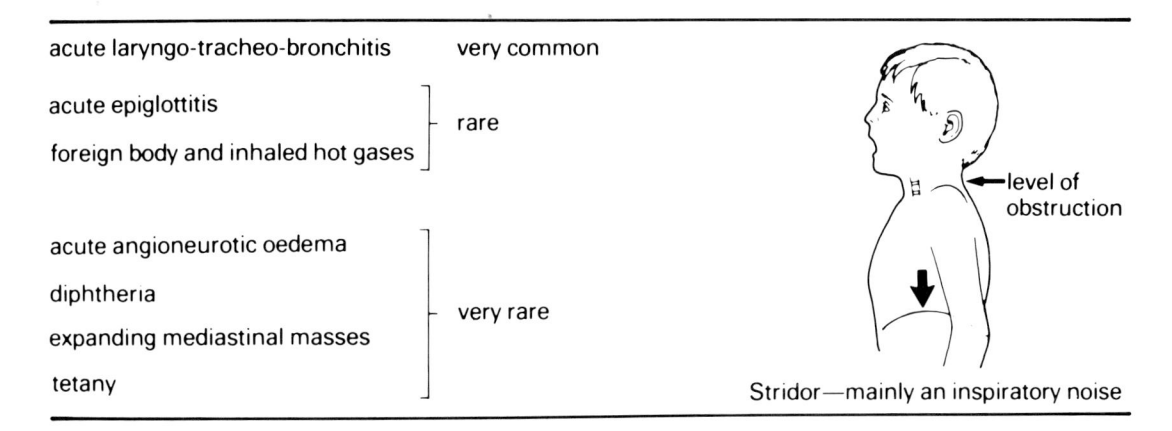

acute laryngo-tracheo-bronchitis	very common	
acute epiglottitis	} rare	
foreign body and inhaled hot gases		← level of obstruction
acute angioneurotic oedema		
diphtheria	} very rare	
expanding mediastinal masses		
tetany		Stridor—mainly an inspiratory noise

Fig. 3.7
Aetiology of stridor (*From Milner AD & Hull D (1984)* Hospital Paediatrics. *Churchill Livingstone, Edinburgh, by courtesy of the publishers*)

signs of clinical deterioration. If stridor becomes so severe that the child is becoming exhausted, then oral intubation followed by nasotracheal intubation performed by a skilled anaesthetist is indicated.

When a diagnosis of epiglottitis is made, elective intubation is arranged because the mortality from an obstructed airway in this condition is high. This infection is caused by *Haemophilus influenzae* infection, so intravenous chloramphenicol is given (at least 10 per cent of these organisms are resistant to ampicillin). Steroids are sometimes given to reduce oedema of the supraglottic area.

Croup is by far the most common cause of stridor in children, and most cases with mild stridor are looked after at home. The morbidity and mortality of stridor are negligible as long as the cases of epiglottitis are recognized and severe croups are observed in hospital.

Laryngomalacia

Luke was taken to his family doctor at 2 months of age with noisy breathing which had been present from 10 days of age. His mother was very concerned and told the doctor that his breathing had been worse during the last few days when he had had a snuffly nose. On questioning it was clear that Luke fed well and was thriving. The noise appeared to cause more worry to the parents than to Luke himself.

When he was examined, a mild inspiratory stridor was present which became worse during crying. The noise was coarse, varied from breath to breath and was changed by different positions of the head. The lungs were clear on auscultation and the chest shape was normal. A diagnosis of laryngomalacia (floppy larynx) was made and the implications explained to the parents.

Comment

This condition is common and is caused by soft laryngeal cartilage which tends to collapse during inspiration. The stridor develops within the first few days of life and persists until about a year when the degree of airway obstruction diminishes. Upper respiratory infections commonly exacerbate the stridor, and severe obstruction can occasionally develop with coexistent croup. When presentation is in the newborn period it is wise to exclude a unilateral choanal atresia by passage of a tube down each nostril in turn.

When typical features of laryngomalacia are present, as in this case, the only investigation indicated is a barium swallow. This will detect an abnormality of the aortic arch or its branches compressing the trachea and oesophagus (vascular ring). Some infants need further investigation by direct laryngoscopy (Table 3.6). With these atypical cases, rare abnormalities such as haemangiomas, webs, cysts or vocal cord palsies will need to be excluded by an ENT surgeon.

The prognosis of laryngomalacia is excellent and full recovery by 3 years is the rule.

Table 3.6

Indications for laryngoscopy in infants with chronic stridor

Severe stridor
Failure to thrive
Chest deformity
Abnormal cry
Persistence of stridor after 3 years

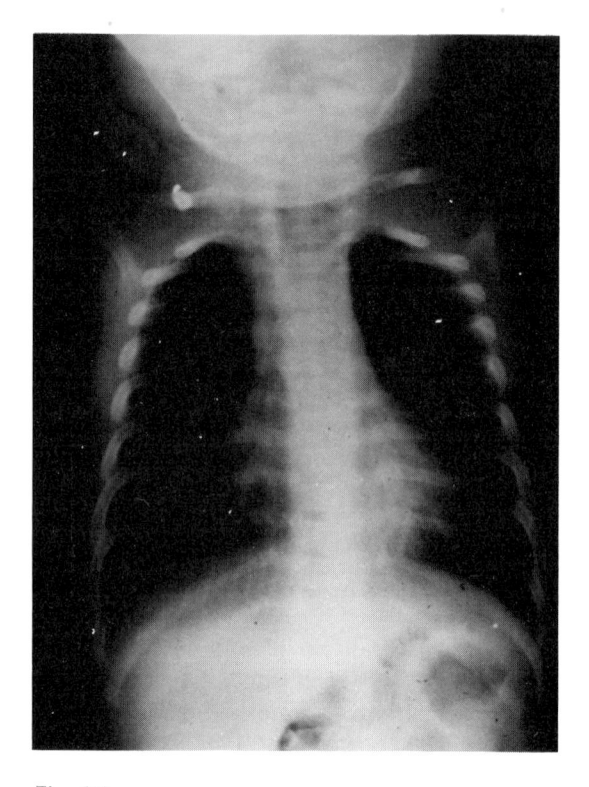

Fig. 3.8
Chest x-ray in bronchiolitis

Bronchiolitis

Daisy, who was nearly 4 months old, developed a cold which was followed 36 hours later by an irritating cough, wheeze and difficulty in feeding. She had been a term baby weighing 3.10 kg and had never been ill before. A fever of 38°C was found as well as rapid wheezy breathing with marked intercostal recession, and a hyperinflated chest. There were also fine crackles audible in most areas towards the end of inspiration, especially at the lung bases.

The chest x-ray (Fig. 3.8) showed hyperinflation with a few small patchy shadows in the upper zones. In view of this clinical picture and x-ray, a nasopharyngeal aspirate was sent for immunofluorescence and revealed the presence of respiratory syncytial virus later that day. In fact, four other infants had been admitted during the previous week with similar findings of acute viral bronchiolitis (Fig. 3.9).

Daisy was sat up in a chair and given two-hourly feeds by a nasogastric tube. Excessive oral secretions were cleared with a mucus extractor and oxygen was administered via a

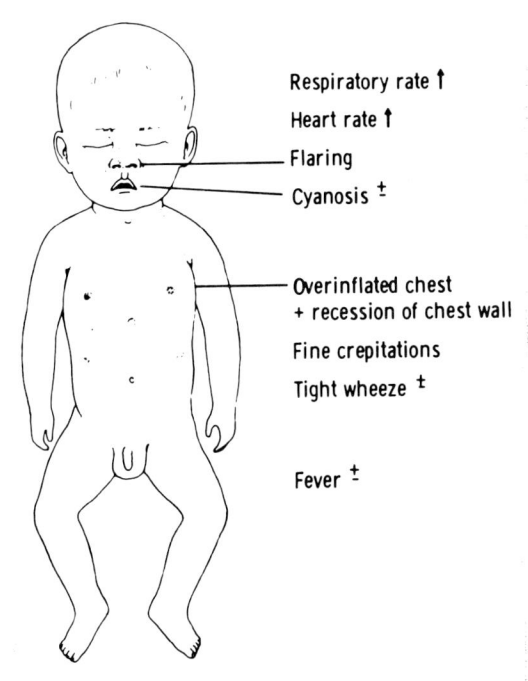

Fig. 3.9
Clinical features of bronchiolitis

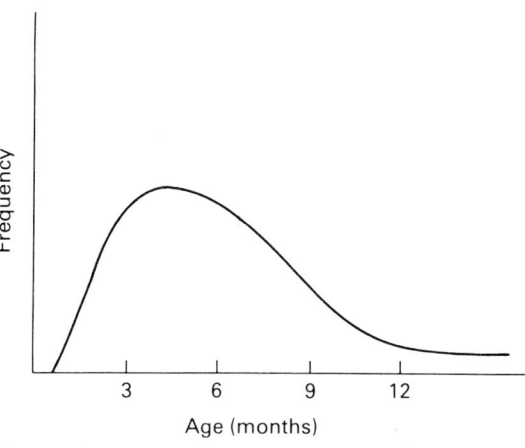

- Respiratory rate ↑
- Heart rate ↑
- Flaring
- Cyanosis ±
- Overinflated chest + recession of chest wall
- Fine crepitations
- Tight wheeze ±
- Fever ±

Fig. 3.10
Age distribution of acute bronchiolitis

headbox. The symptoms settled over the next six days and Daisy was discharged home after a week.

Comment

Acute bronchiolitis results from necrosis of the epithelial lining of the terminal bronchioles, secondary to viral colonization, usually by respiratory syncytial virus which is found in over 80 per cent of cases. The infection most commonly presents at 3–6 months of age (Fig. 3.10), during the winter months when epidemics occur.

Asthma can be confused with bronchiolitis but the absence of fine crackles, age over 9 months and the summer presentation favour the former. Bronchopneumonia causes more constitutional disturbance without wheezing and the chest x-ray shows consolidation.

The management of bronchiolitis is supportive, needing high standards of nursing care (Table 3.7). No drug other than oxygen significantly alters the course of the disease. Fewer

Table 3.7
Management of bronchiolitis

Sit up
Nasogastric tube feeds
Intravenous fluids if particularly ill
Clear mouth of secretions
Oxygen if cyanosed
Careful observation of colour, respiratory rate and pattern of breathing

than 1 per cent of infants will need mechanical ventilation, and arterial blood gas measurements which show progressive respiratory failure and exhaustion will favour this course of action. The majority of infants have fully recovered by seven to ten days, but long-term studies show persisting abnormalities on lung function tests and there is a high incidence of asthma in later years.

Whooping Cough

Tom was admitted to hospital at 5 months with a ten-day history of episodes of paroxysmal coughing followed by vomiting. His 3-year-old sister had developed an intermittent cough three weeks before this. The coughing bouts were seen by the nursing staff who witnessed about eight to ten episodes each day, lasting a minute or so and associated with intense congestion of the face and cyanosis. There was no whoop after the coughing paroxysms. Tom had received his first immunization at 3 months against diphtheria, tetanus and polio, but the whooping cough vaccine had been omitted because of the parents' concern about side effects.

Tom's examination was unremarkable and a chest x-ray was normal. His blood count revealed a lymphocytosis of $35 \times 10^9/l$ and a pernasal swab grew *Bordetella pertussis*. Careful observations were carried out and a course of erythromycin given. During the next few days his feeding deteriorated and he became rather listless so he was transferred to the children's intensive care unit. His general condition worsened over the next few hours with increasingly severe paroxysms, so intravenous rather than oral fluids were given. His downhill course continued so that he became semiconscious, responding only when handled. Respiratory failure was excluded by a normal chest x-ray and blood gas analysis, and a lumbar puncture was normal. He stopped breathing shortly afterwards, but in spite of mechanical ventilation and intravenous antibiotics he died later that day. A post-mortem showed widespread petechial haemorrhages throughout the brain and evidence of anoxic damage.

Comment

Whooping cough epidemics appear every four years and during the 1950s up to 60 000 cases were notified every three months in England and Wales (Fig. 3.11). The introduction of immunization in 1957 reduced these numbers but recent adverse publicity against the vaccine reduced uptake to about 30 per cent during the early 1980s, and resulted in a large epidemic. There are 10–20 deaths a year from whooping cough and nearly all these are in children under 1 year of age, who develop respiratory failure secondary to lung collapse or brain damage from anoxia and haemorrhage.

The typical clinical features of the illness are secondary to damage to the epithelial lining of the respiratory tract and production of tenacious mucus (Table 3.8). Treatment is supportive, with careful monitoring by nursing staff.

Table 3.8

Clinical features of whooping cough

Incubation period	10–14 days
Catarrhal stage	Cough and runny nose for 1 week
Paroxysmal stage	Paroxysmal cough for 2–8 weeks
	Inspiratory whoop
	Congestion of the face
	Cyanosis
	Apnoea
	Vomiting

No drug has been shown to have any definite beneficial effect on outcome, but steroids, phenobarbitone and salbutamol are sometimes tried.

Prevention is by immunization, which, although not totally effective, reduces the risk of disease. The incidence of neurological sequelae to the vaccine is about 1 in 300 000, but the risk of brain damage following the disease is unknown. Immunization should be offered to all children as long as there is no specific contraindication (Table 3.9). Prophy-

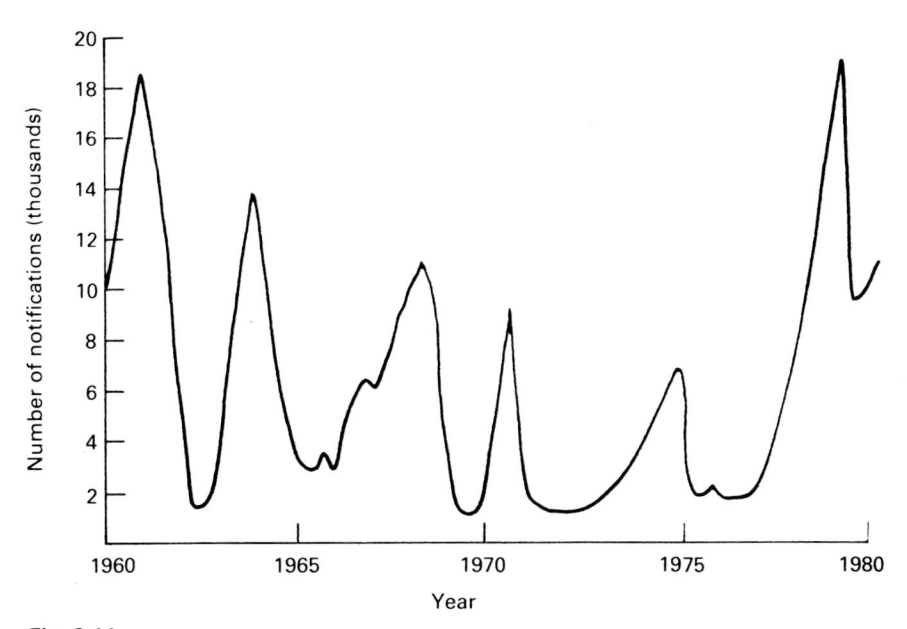

Fig. 3.11
Quarterly whooping cough notifications for England and Wales 1960–1980

lactic erythromycin or contrimoxazole given during the incubation period of the disease are effective in preventing some cases, and there is some evidence that erythromycin in the first few days of the illness foreshortens the course of the disease.

Table 3.9

Contraindications to whooping cough immunization

Absolute
A severe reaction (local or systemic) to a previous dose of triple vaccine

Relative
A history of epilepsy in the child, parents or siblings
A history of continuing neurological problems

Temporary
An intercurrent infection with fever (not just a cough or a runny nose)

Whooping cough is once again common due to undermining of the immunization programme. The occasional death from the disease is a preventable tragedy.

Asthma

Anna, a 9-year-old asthmatic, was reviewed in the outpatient clinic (Fig. 3.12). Her father had brought her along because her mother was housebound in a wheelchair with advanced multiple sclerosis. Anna's only sibling, a 6-year-old brother, was well apart from occasional episodes of 'bronchitis' which appeared to be related to colds.

During recent months, Anna had been missing a lot of school because of coughing or wheezing bouts. Her father and the teaching staff did not get on well together, and there were problems about the use of inhalers at school. Anna's symptoms were mainly exacerbated by emotional upsets at home.

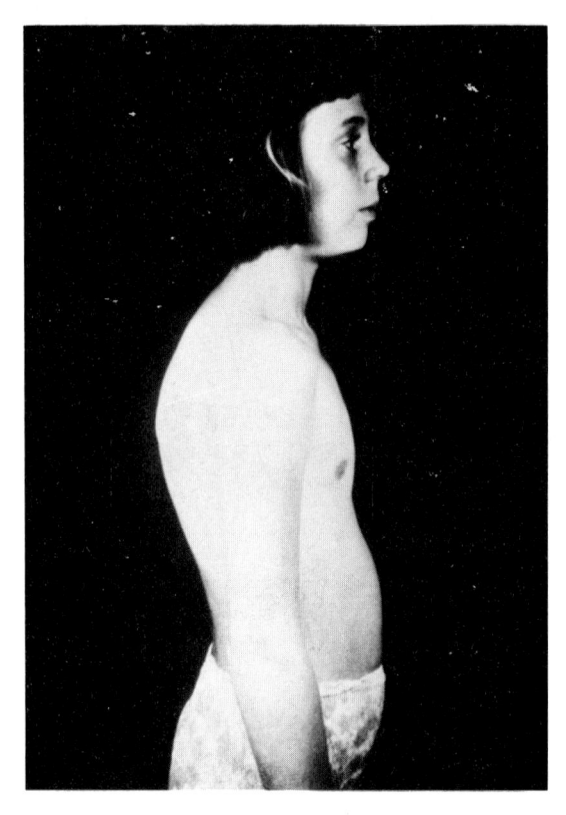

Fig. 3.12
Chest deformity in chronic asthma

Sodium cromoglycate by spinhaler and a salbutamol inhaler had been used for the last year and were given three times each day, but compliance had been poor.

The chest x-ray showed gross hyperinflation with flat diaphragms and a bulging sternum on the lateral film consistent with the clinical appearance (Fig. 3.13). Her peak flow was 85 litres per minute (expected for height 120–280 litres per minute) (Fig. 3.14).

In view of the treatment failure, cromoglycate was stopped, replaced by regular beclomethasone by inhaler four times a day and the dose of salbutamol was increased with advice given about its use prior to exercise or sport. A course of oral prednisolone was also started, tailing off over a few days to provide maximum initial impact. The health visitor was contacted to liaise with the school, family and general practitioner.

Anna's symptoms did not change very much with these new measures and the severity of symptoms appeared to be closely related to tension at home.

Comment

Asthma is one of the commonest childhood illnesses. Studies in general practice reveal that one in five children will have one or more wheezing attacks during the first ten years of life. The diagnosis is frequently missed (as in Anna's brother) when the main symptom is persistent cough, characteristically worse at night. The inappropriate label of 'bronchitis' tends to lead to multiple courses of antibiotics when bronchodilator therapy would be more appropriate.

Anna's asthma as judged by chest deformity, chest x-ray and peak flow was severe. Although she had never been admitted to hospital, it was apparent that she had limitations in most of the everyday activities that children of her age take for granted. A course of oral steroids is useful in this situation as the dramatic improvement that follows reveals to the family the severity of the disease. Long-term oral steroids are best avoided because of complications such as growth failure and Cushing's syndrome. There are several suitable drugs for asthma prophylaxis (Table 3.10), but the young child will need to use a device such as a Rotahaler if the drug is to be inhaled.

Emotional and psychological upsets are often associated with severe asthma. It is generally possible for asthmatic children to attend normal schools, but on rare occasions placement in a residential school (so-called

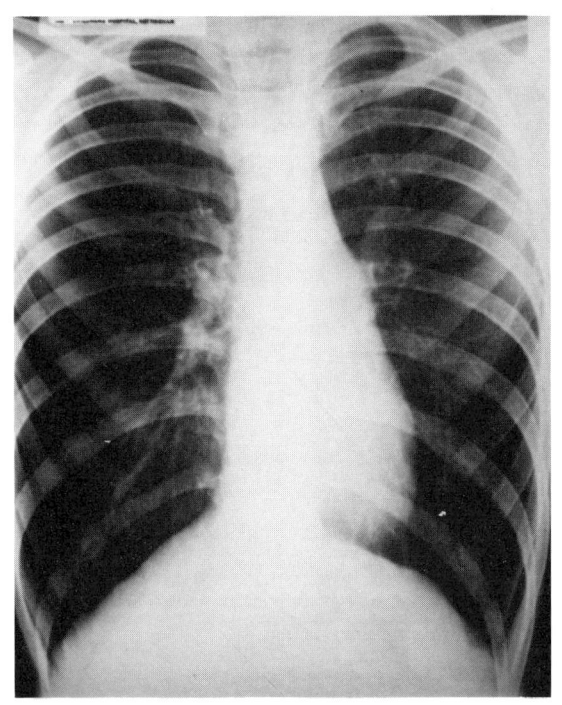

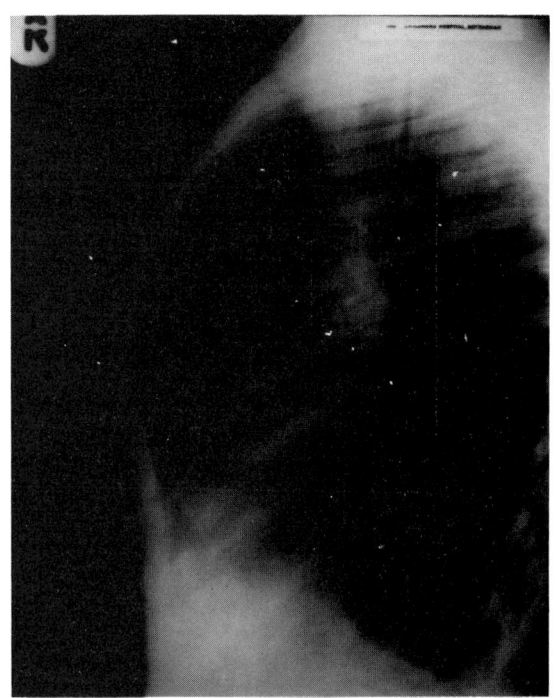

Fig. 3.13
Chest x-rays in asthma

'parentectomy') may be desirable. Sometimes limited success in the management of chronic illness must be accepted and the temptation for the enthusiast to inflict treatment worse than the disease should be resisted! Seven out of ten children will grow out of their asthma by 12 years, but the severity of Anna's disease makes this unlikely in her case.

Tuberculosis

Khalid, a 10-year-old boy of Pakistani parents, had been unwell with vague symptoms over the previous few months, the most prominent being sweating at night. His father, who owned a restaurant business, had been in hospital for two weeks and was found to have

Table 3.10

Drug prophylaxis in asthma

	Nebulizer (under 4 years)	Powder inhaler (4–10 years)	Aerosol inhaler (over 10 years)	Oral (any age)
Sodium cromoglycate	√	√	√	—
Beclomethasone	√	√	√	√
Theophylline	—	—	—	√
Salbutamol (before exercise)	√	√	√	√
Ipratropium bromide	√	—	√	—

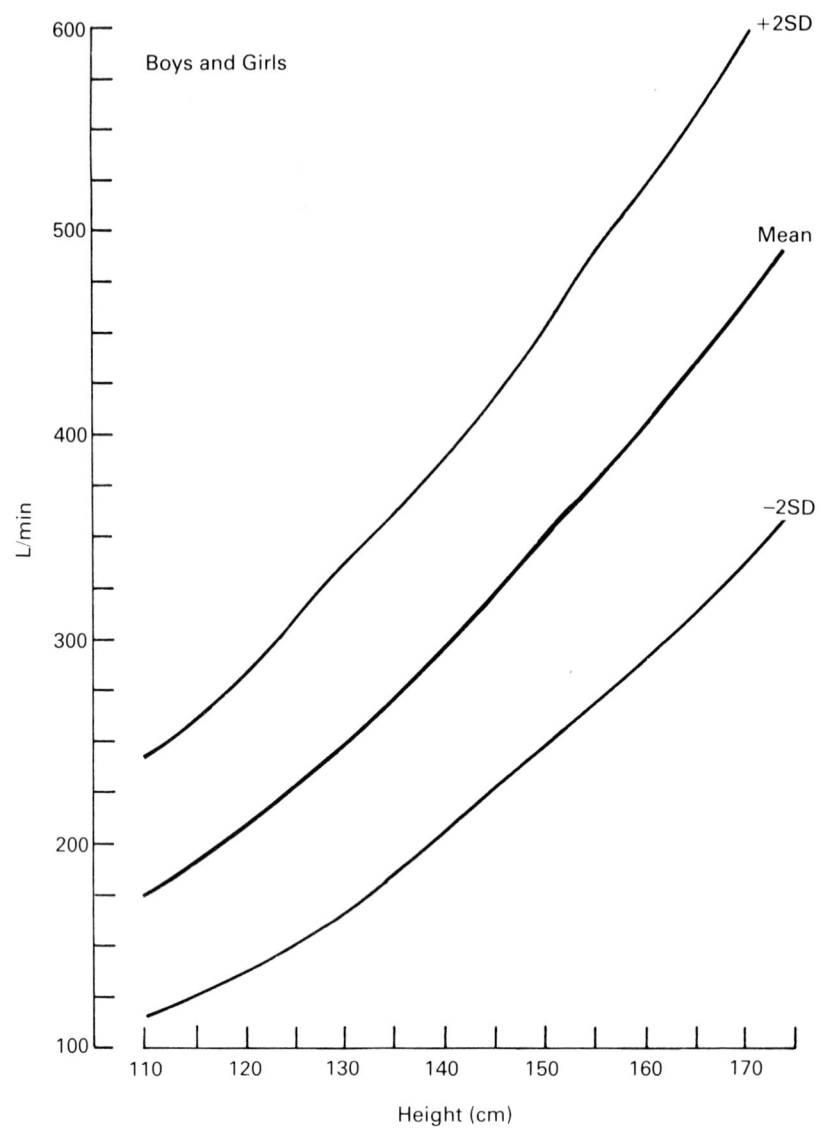

Fig. 3.14
Predicted peak flow measurements in children

open pulmonary tuberculosis. Khalid had a positive Heaf test and an abnormal chest x-ray (Fig. 3.15) showing an elevated right diaphragm, right-sided hilar nodes and extensive shadowing of the right mid zone, extending out from the hilum. The lateral film showed extensive collapse in the lower part of the right upper lobe.

Khalid's disease was notified, and the environmental health officer closed the family business for two weeks until the rest of the family had been screened. Triple therapy was

RESPIRATORY DISEASES 33

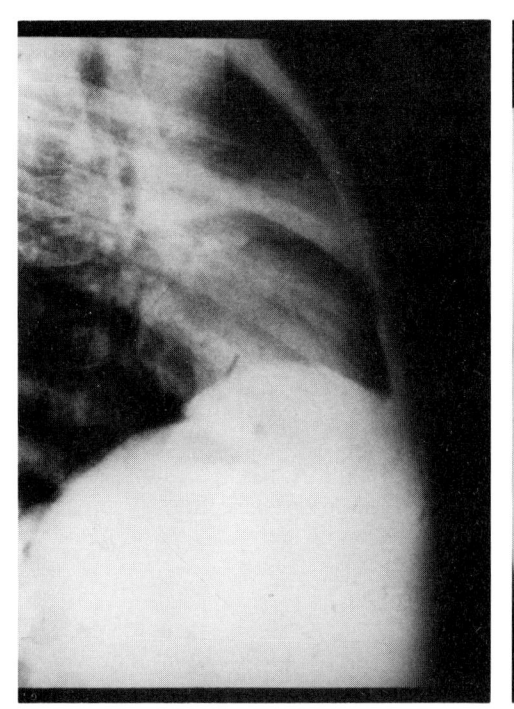

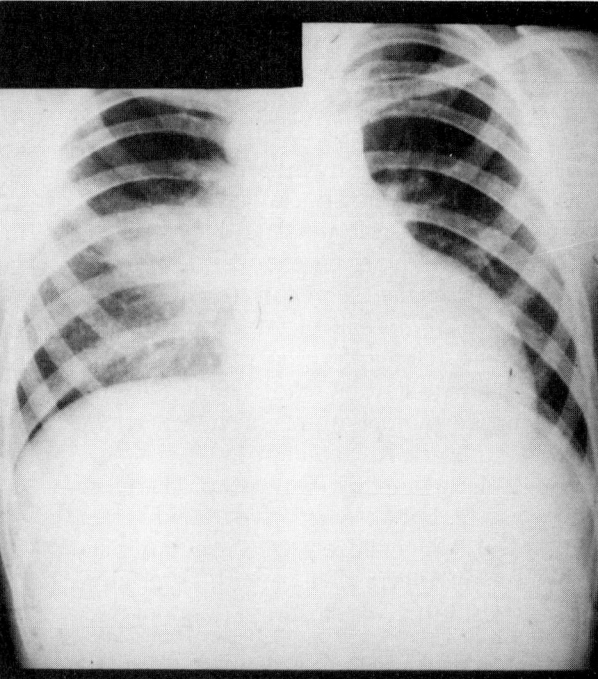

Fig. 3.15
Chest x-rays in pulmonary tuberculosis

given (rifampicin, isoniazid and ethambutol), with careful monitoring of urine samples to ensure compliance with the nine-month treatment schedule. There was gradual resolution of Khalid's symptoms.

Comment

Tuberculosis is still relatively common in the Asian community. Over all, only 10 per cent of children at the age of 12 have a positive Heaf test in the UK. The primary focus, often in the lung or tonsil, is generally tiny, and the regional lymph nodes in the mediastinum (Fig. 3.16) or neck become secondarily enlarged and caseous. In children the pulmonary problems are secondary to obstruction of a bronchus, leading to collapse/consolidation, or leading to emphy-

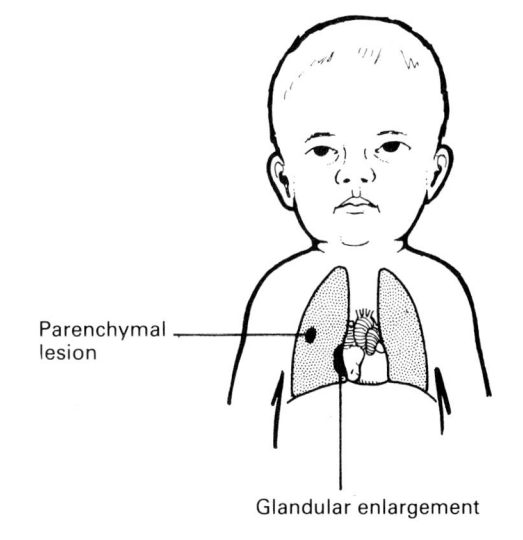

Fig. 3.16
Illustration of primary complex in tuberculosis

sema due to a ball-valve effect. Pleural effusions also occur. Sometimes the disease may become apparent within a few weeks of the initial contact, with the development of erythema nodosum.

Symptoms vary greatly in primary tuberculosis. Many children appear asymptomatic, whereas others are febrile, ill and lose a great deal of weight. The main concern during the first year of the disease in children is the risk of blood stream spread of infection, leading to the dreaded complication of tuberculous meningitis or miliary spread. The latter may be diagnosed by looking at the fundi, when choroidal tubercles are sometimes seen.

Tuberculin testing by Mantoux or Heaf test is very useful, but false negative tests do arise (Table 3.11). In children with pneumonias which are slow to resolve or with atypical x-ray features, tuberculin testing is mandatory.

Table 3.11

Causes of false negative tuberculin tests

Fulminating miliary spread of the disease
Intercurrent viral infection such as measles
Steroid therapy
Malnutrition

Control of infection involves prevention by BCG immunization (Table 3.12), treatment of 'open' adult disease, which is infectious, and tracing of family contacts which is arranged by liaison with the chest physician. Modern drugs have shortened treatment courses from 18 months to 9 months but combination therapy is still given to prevent the development of drug resistance.

The prognosis is excellent in nearly all cases of tuberculosis in children except following meningitis where there is a high risk of permanent brain damage. Surgical removal of a col-

Table 3.12

BCG immunization

BCG immunization is indicated for:
School children at the age of 12 years with a negative Heaf test
Newborn infants of Asian families
Household contacts of active case (if Heaf negative)
Nurses and other health service workers (if Heaf negative)

lapsed lobe which fails to expand or develops bronchiectasis is rarely needed.

Pneumonia

Carl, a 5 year old, had been unwell for 24 hours with fever, upper abdominal pain and occasional coughing. He was usually a healthy child who had received all his routine immunizations and was now 'growing out' of breath-holding attacks which had been a problem during the previous year. When examined he looked poorly, was pyrexial with a temperature of 39.4°C, and had a respiratory rate of 44 per minute. There was dullness to percussion at the base of the left chest, and bronchial breathing with a few fine crackles audible over this area on auscultation. A diagnosis of pneumonia was made and the parents were specifically questioned to exclude a history of foreign body inhalation.

The chest x-ray showed extensive consolidation of the middle and lower zones of the left lung (Fig. 3.17). Following a throat swab and blood culture, Carl was commenced on intravenous benzylpenicillin. His symptoms settled over 36 hours and coarse crackles developed, indicating resolution. The blood cultures and throat swabs failed to grow any pathogens.

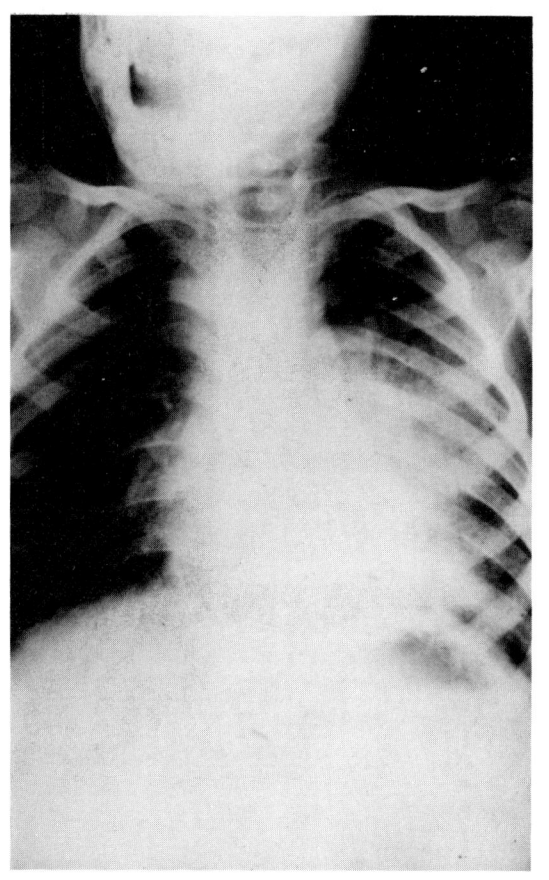

Fig. 3.17
Chest x-ray in pneumonia

Comment

Pneumonia causing inflammatory consolidation of alveoli or infiltration of interstitial tissues is common in children, especially those under 3 years. With extensive pneumonia, generalized signs will strongly suggest the diagnosis before the chest itself is examined (Fig. 3.18).

Many chest infections in children are caused by viruses (Table 3.13) and the illness may follow an upper respiratory infection. In this situation the only signs may be a few localized fine crackles, but an x-ray is likely to show a patchy bronchopneumonia over a wider area. The pneumococcus is the commonest bacteria causing pneumonia, tending to produce involvement of one lobe. Occasionally more than one lobe is affected, as in Carl's case. About 40 per cent will have a positive blood culture but bacteriological diagnosis in individual cases may be impossible, as throat swabs tend to grow commensals.

It is recommended that antibiotics be used for all pneumonias, as the viral and bacterial ones cannot be separated with certainty. In children under a year who are very toxic and sick, the possibility of staphylococcal pneumonia should be considered, and in children between 5 and 15 years with symptoms slow

Table 3.13

Agents causing pneumonia in children

Viruses	
Respiratory syncytial virus } Parainfluenza virus	In infants and young children
Mycoplasma	The commonest cause of pneumonia in school children
Bacteria	
Pneumococcus	All ages (common)
Haemophilus influenzae	In young children (uncommon)
Staphylococcus aureus	In infants (uncommon)

36 CLINICAL CASES IN PAEDIATRICS

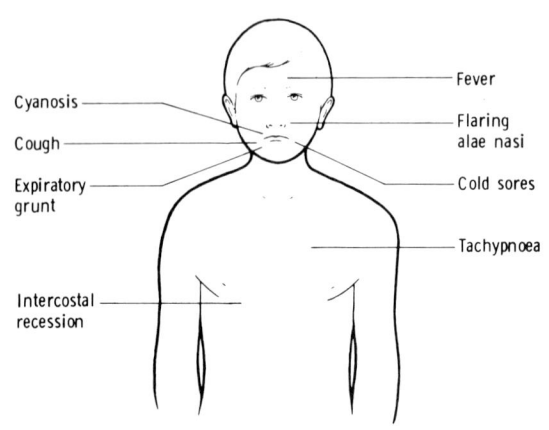

Fig. 3.18
Generalized signs of pneumonia

to settle, mycoplasma infection is a possibility. Physiotherapy is probably best reserved for cases of delayed resolution.

The prognosis is excellent unless there is pre-existing disease, although staphylococcal pneumonia can be fatal in infants. If there is delayed resolution the possibility of other pathology such as cystic fibrosis or foreign body should be considered. In developing countries, pneumonia (often viral) is the most common cause of death after infective diarrhoea.

Cystic Fibrosis

John, who was 12 years old, presented shortly after birth with meconium ileus. An erect abdominal x-ray (Fig. 3.19) revealed absence of gas in the bowel distally, but dilation of the stomach and upper small bowel. A successful laparotomy at 12 hours of age relieved his bowel obstruction. The diagnosis of cystic fibrosis was confirmed at 8 weeks by a diagnostic sweat test (Fig. 3.20) where sweating was stimulated by pilocarpine iontophoresis. The sweat sodium and chloride were 79 mmol/l (values above 60 mmol/l are diag-

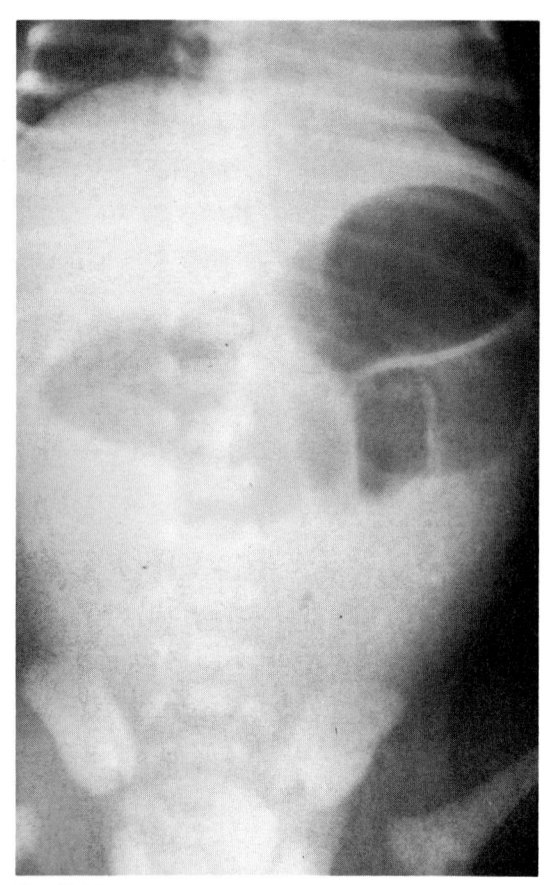

Fig. 3.19
X-ray showing meconium ileus

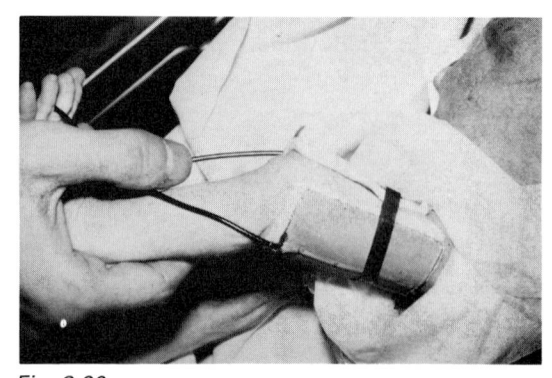

Fig. 3.20
Sweat test

nostic as long as more than 100 mg of sweat is collected).

John's mother had been concerned with his general condition for two weeks and had brought him up to clinic earlier than expected. He had had poor appetite and a low grade fever associated with increasing cough, sputum production and breathlessness. She commented that John 'looked blue around the lips'. Examination confirmed this, as well as the finding of finger clubbing. John was thin with gross muscle wasting and had a barrel-shaped chest (Fig. 3.21). There were generalized wheezes present in all areas of his chest, with bilateral coarse crackles audible at both lung bases.

Comment

Although the lungs are normal at birth, repeated episodes of infection and obstruction of small airways with viscous secretions damage the lungs. Children are often relatively well until a lower respiratory tract infection causes an exacerbation of symptoms. Two viral infections that cause further lung damage, measles and influenza, can be prevented by immunization.

John's chest x-ray showed hyperinflation, hilar gland enlargement and patchy shadowing which was especially prominent in the right lower zone (Fig. 3.22). His older brother,

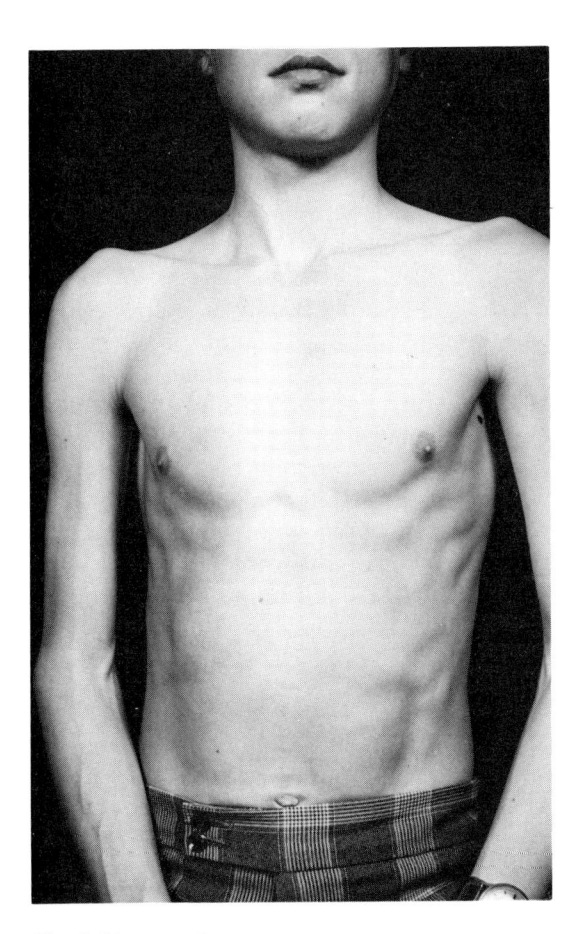

Fig. 3.21
Child with cystic fibrosis

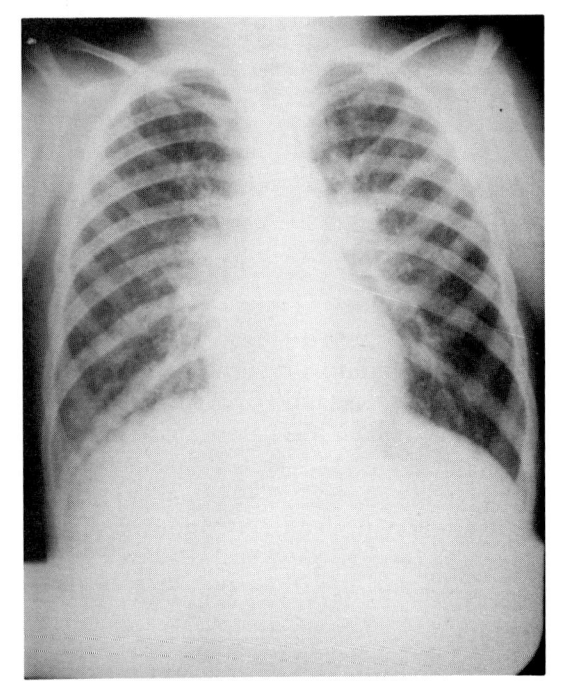

Fig. 3.22
Chest x-ray in early cystic fibrosis

Matthew with advanced cystic fibrosis, has irreversible lung damage with gross hyperinflation and more extensive shadowing (Fig. 3.23).

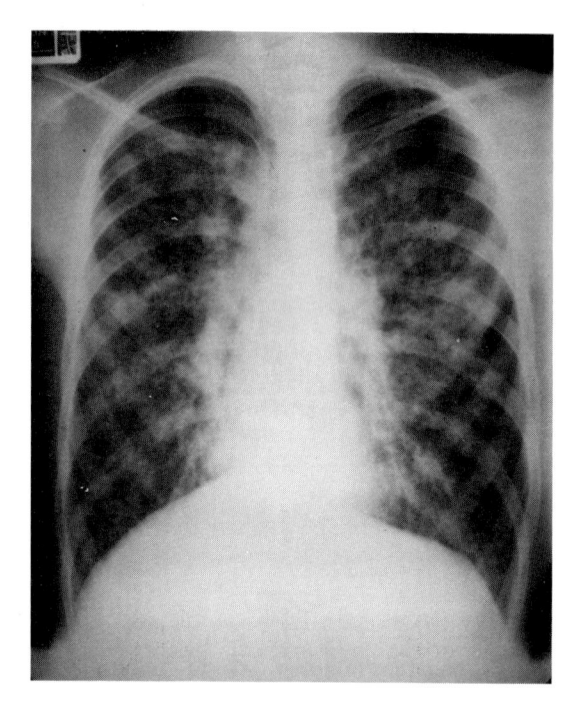

Fig. 3.23
Chest x-ray in advanced cystic fibrosis

The commonest bacterial pathogens in the lungs of children with cystic fibrosis are *Staphylococcus aureus* and *Haemophilus influenzae*. When there have been repeated courses of antibiotics, *Pseudomonas aeruginosa* tends to colonize the sputum. This organism is rarely fully eradicated, even with appropriate antibiotics. John was given a three-week course of amoxycillin, as his last sputum had grown *H. influenzae*. His mother was given further instruction in chest physiotherapy using postural drainage three times daily (Fig. 3.24) and his symptoms rapidly subsided over the next week.

Since almost all children with cystic fibrosis have malabsorption due to pancreatic insufficiency, oral pancreatic and vitamin supplements are necessary. Further essential management will include support of the family and contact with the Cystic Fibrosis Trust. Genetic counselling is needed for this recessively inherited disease. It is one of the commonest inherited diseases in Caucasians, with a frequency of 1 in 2200, and it has been suggested that early treatment improves the prognosis. For these reasons, attempts have been made to develop a screening test for neonatal use; blood trypsin levels are currently under investigation. Survival and quality of life have improved over the last 30 years with more intensive treatment and some children are now surviving to early adult life.

Foreign Body Inhalation

Darren, a 3 year old, was seen in the accident and emergency department on a Sunday afternoon with an irritating cough and wheeze which had started a few days before. He had not had any chest troubles in the past, and there was no family history of asthma. School had finished for half term so the family were due to go away on holiday the next morning. The parents wanted some antibiotic for Darren to take during his week in the Isle of Wight.

On examination, air entry to the right side of the chest was reduced with widespread wheezes audible, more marked on the right than the left side of the chest. In view of these findings the casualty officer went back over the history with the parents. Apparently six days prior to this visit to the accident and emergency department, Darren had had a choking episode whilst eating a handful of peanuts. He had been unable to breathe for a few seconds and had become very red in

RESPIRATORY DISEASES 39

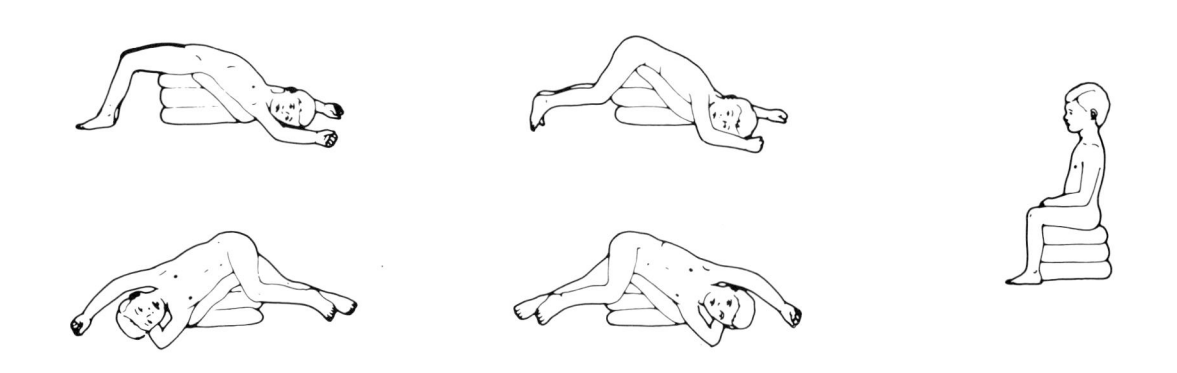

Fig. 3.24
Postural drainage techniques

the face. After a coughing spell, his symptoms rapidly disappeared.

Chest x-rays were taken at the end of inspiration and expiration. The former was normal but the expiratory film (Fig. 3.25) showed some mediastinal shift to the left with emphysema of the right lung. Darren was admitted to hospital and a bronchoscopy was carried out the next morning at which a peanut was removed from the right main bronchus (Fig. 3.26). A few days later a postcard from the Isle of Wight reported that the holiday was a success in spite of the two-day delay!

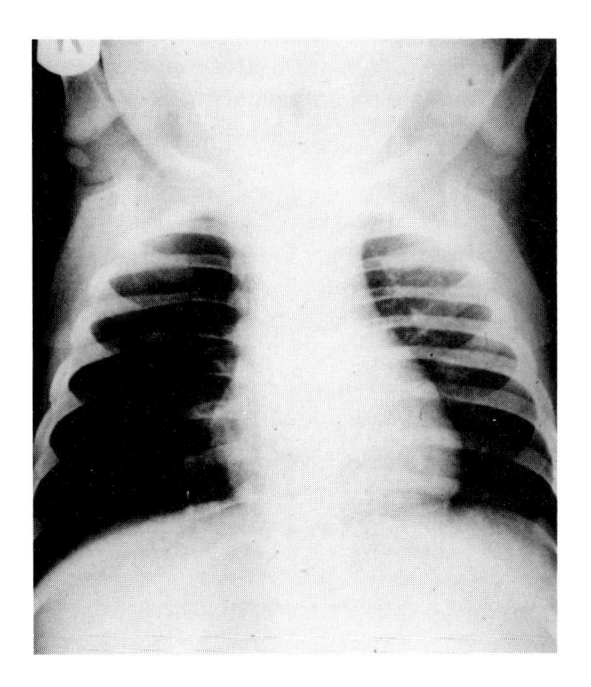

Fig. 3.25
Chest x-ray in foreign body inhalation

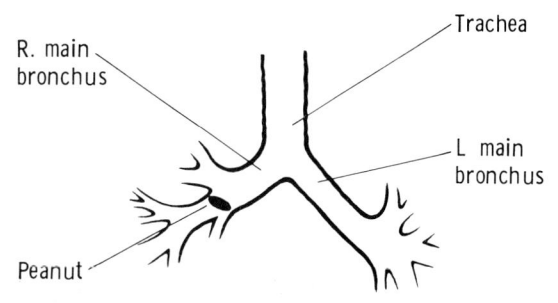

Fig. 3.26
Diagram of obstruction to right main bronchus

Comment

The majority of children who inhale foreign bodies are under 4 years old, and, as with most accidents, boys are more commonly involved. Peanuts are the most frequently inhaled object but toys or pieces of plastic such as pen-tops are commonly found. Unfortunately, the majority of foreign bodies are radiolucent.

Most foreign bodies lodge in a mainstem bronchus, particularly the right bronchus since this has a more vertical course. Larger foreign bodies can obstruct the larynx. Sudden death from choking from a food bolus occurs in about 300 people each year in the UK. The Heimlich manoeuvre—a sudden firm squeeze over the epigastrium in an inward and upward direction—will generally eject the bolus.

With intrabronchial foreign bodies, ball-valve obstruction causes overinflation initially before infection and lung collapse supervene. Late presentation after several weeks of an intrabronchial foreign body can result in extensive lung damage, and the bronchogram of such a child reveals extensive bronchiectasis of the left lower lobe (Fig. 3.27).

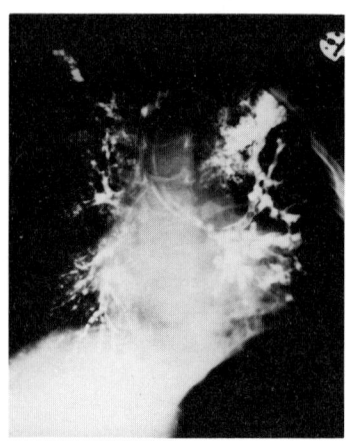

Fig. 3.27
Bronchogram showing bronchiectasis

Bronchoscopy will enable a diagnosis to be made and will usually allow removal of the offending object. Intensive physiotherapy and antibiotics should lead to full resolution unless permanent lung damage has been sustained.

4 Cardiovascular diseases

Supraventricular Tachycardia

Daniel, a 3 month old, presented with a 12-hour history of pallor, breathlessness and poor feeding. He had previously been fit and was thriving normally. An anxious expression was noted on his face and he looked ill, with a respiratory rate of 70 per minute and marked intercostal recession. Chest examination revealed fine basal crackles and his liver was palpable 5 cm below the costal margin. His pulse was rapid and weak, with a rate in excess of 200 per minute, and impossible to count accurately. The heart sounds were indistinguishable from each other and no murmurs were heard.

An electrocardiogram (ECG) was performed at the standard speed of 25 mm per second (Fig. 4.1). It showed a rapid, regular

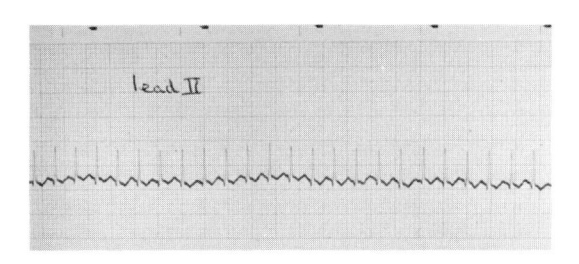

Fig. 4.1
ECG of supraventricular tachycardia

rhythm of 320 per minute with normal QRS complexes and absent P waves. The features of Daniel's illness are summarized in Fig. 4.2. These are the findings of supraventricular tachycardia (SVT), and the most common

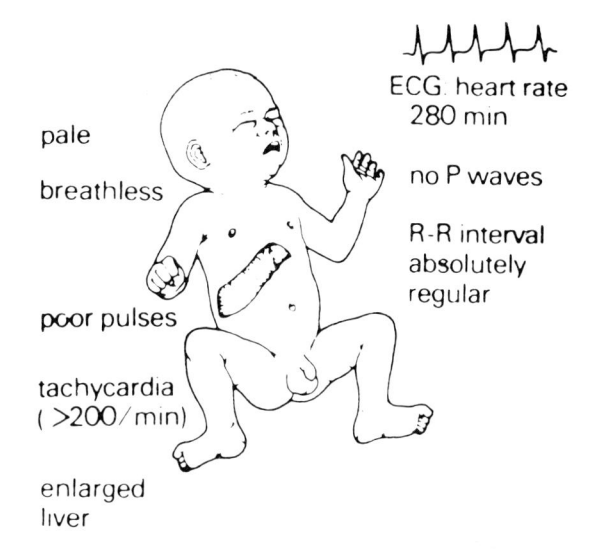

Fig. 4.2
Clinical features of supraventricular tachycardia (*From Milner AD & Hull D (1984)* Hospital Paediatrics. *Churchill Livingstone, Edinburgh, by courtesy of the publishers*)

mechanism is shown in Fig. 4.3, with predisposing causes listed in Table 4.1.

Daniel's chest x-ray showed an enlarged heart, with mottled shadowing radiating out from the hila and relative sparing of the periphery—the typical features of pulmonary oedema. His enlarged liver confirmed that congestive heart failure secondary to the tachycardia was present.

The first line of treatment is vagal stimulation, and is best carried out with the child attached to an ECG monitor. Either the

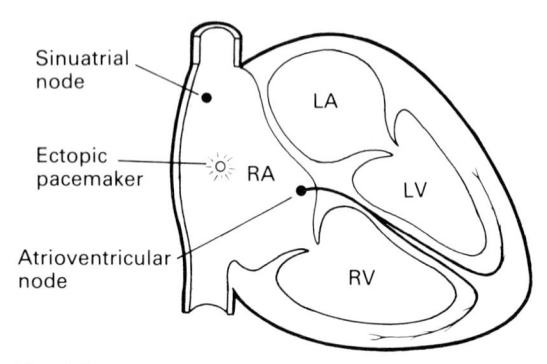

Fig. 4.3
Ectopic pacemaker in supraventricular tachycardia

Table 4.1

Causes of supraventricular tachycardia in childhood

A febrile illness, particularly pneumonia
Accidental poisoning, particularly with tricyclic antidepressants
Wolff–Parkinson–White syndrome (an accessory conducting pathway between the atria and ventricles)
Unknown (the majority)

Table 4.2

Vagal stimulation in children with SVT

Young children and infants	Diving reflex (application of an ice pack or cold flannel to the face)
Older children	Eyeball pressure Carotid sinus massage Valsalva manoeuvre Swallowing a mouthful of ice cream

rhythm reverts to normal or it does not work at all (Table 4.2). Unfortunately, these measures were not successful.

Because he was unwell and in cardiac failure, Daniel was sat up and given oxygen. Intravenous frusemide was given with dramatic improvement in his symptoms. A loading dose of digoxin was given orally (peak plasma levels are reached in 60 minutes) with no change in heart rate over the next two hours. However, he suddenly reverted to sinus rhythm in the next hour with a rate of 140 per minute.

Comment

There were no recurrences of his tachycardia and the parents were given an excellent prognosis. Older children and those with the Wolff–Parkinson–White syndrome are more liable to recurrences and may need prophylactic drugs (digoxin or a beta blocker). Treatment of the very ill child requires the use of DC shock. Occasionally, SVT may be intermittent and difficult to diagnose, in which case a 24-hour ECG tape recording at home may be helpful.

Innocent Murmur

Jane, an 8 year old, was the only child of parents in their mid forties. Her father was a jeweller and her mother was a housewife. Jane had had recurrent upper respiratory infections during the preceding year, which caused much worry as a heart murmur had been discovered. Since a family friend had rheumatic fever as a child leading to mitral stenosis, Jane's mother was keen for Jane to have antibiotics for all febrile illnesses.

A confrontation developed between Jane's mother and the head teacher at school over swimming, as the school wanted a doctor's letter before permanently excusing Jane from this activity. None seemed to be forthcoming, so Jane was assessed by the school medical officer (with the parents' permission!)

A systolic murmur was heard in the second intercostal space just lateral to the sternal border. It was midsystolic in timing and grade 2 in intensity (out of 6), and nearly disappeared in the supine position. The heart sounds appeared normal, as was the rest of the examination, so the doctor thought that these were the typical features of an innocent murmur (Table 4.3). Because of parental

Table 4.3
Features of an innocent murmur

Low intensity
Heard over a limited area
Midsystolic (except venous hum)
Short
Musical, buzzing, vibratory quality
Absence of cardiac symptoms
No other signs of heart disease

anxiety, a second opinion was arranged at which the physical signs were confirmed and investigations (ECG and x-ray) were normal. A long discussion was held with the family to explain that Jane's heart was normal.

Comment

Heart murmurs are found in up to 96 per cent of children between 3 and 14 years when checked by cardiologists with good hearing. Fortunately these noises are generally soft and difficult for most of us to hear. Since a heart murmur is the commonest presenting feature of congenital heart disease, accurate diagnosis is essential. Certainly the character of the murmur and the absence of other signs usually enable the examiner to be confident in classifying a murmur as innocent. Nevertheless, some relatively loud murmurs can be very difficult to distinguish, even for a cardiologist, so where there is doubt it is wise to refer for a second opinion. For the inexperienced examiner the nature of the second heart sound may be difficult to determine—is the splitting of the aortic and pulmonary components normal, or is it fixed in inspiration and expiration? A fixed split will indicate an atrial septal defect.

Another form of murmur commonly found in children is a venous hum produced by turbulent blood in the major veins as they enter the thorax. It is heard under the clavicles and can be quite loud. It may initially be confused with patent ductus arteriosus, as the murmur may be present in both systole and diastole. However, a venous hum can easily be distinguished because the murmur disappears on lying down.

Cardiac neurosis in a child can be devastating when restrictions on everyday activities such as exercise and sport are imposed. Guilt feelings may lead to overprotection, and so the child is rejected by his peers as being 'different' or as unable to participate in play. Good communications between doctor and family should prevent this tragedy occurring.

Patent Ductus Arteriosus

Brett, aged 6 months, was seen because of failure to thrive. He was born weighing 3.10 kg, but now his weight was on the 3rd centile and length on the 50th centile for age. Brett's mother was unmarried and had two other children aged 4 and 6 years and the family lived in a damp two-bedroomed flat. Attempts at rehousing had been unsuccessful in spite of help from a social worker, as the rent was always several months in arrears. Brett's chest infections over the last three months and failure to thrive had been put down to environmental causes.

At examination, Brett was thin but alert and

responsive. His liver was enlarged to 5 cm below the costal margin, although his spleen was not palpable. He had bounding pulses and a clinically enlarged heart with a marked precordial impulse. The pulmonary component of the second heart sound was moderately loud, and a 'machinery' murmur (a harsh murmur of irregular intensity and low pitch), which was continuous throughout the cardiac cycle, was audible under the left clavicle (Fig. 4.4).

The chest x-ray showed an enlarged heart (more than half the diameter of the chest). The lung fields were plethoric, indicating an increased pulmonary blood flow. Brett had a patent ductus arteriosus (PDA) of moderate size (Fig. 4.5). The duct was ligated and transected at surgery, and this procedure was uneventful (Fig. 4.6).

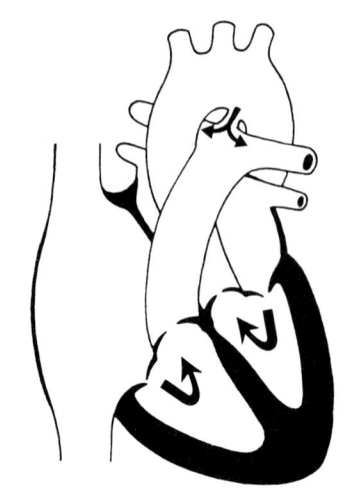

Fig. 4.5
Diagram of patent ductus arteriosus

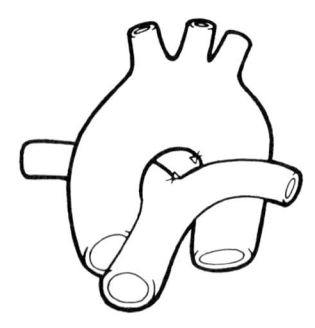

Fig. 4.6
Division of patent ductus arteriosus

Machinery murmur — radiates through to back

Collapsing pulses

ECG – left ventricular hypertrophy (LVH)

Chest x-ray – cardiomegaly, pulmonary plethora

Fig. 4.4
Patent ductus arteriosus

Comment

The ductus arteriosus closes by 15 hours in the normal term baby. Patent ductus arteriosus is commonly found in preterm babies of less than 32 weeks' gestation and has been estimated to occur in up to 40 per cent of infants weighing less than 1.50 kg. It may complicate neonatal respiratory problems but will generally close spontaneously by 3 months. The high incidence of PDA makes it one of the commonest congenital heart lesions. The incidence is 30 times greater in children living at altitudes of more than 5000 m. Although generally an isolated condition, it may occur in conjunction with other heart lesions.

In the preterm baby a PDA may be closed by administration of a prostaglandin inhibitor such as indomethacin. The corollary of this is that a deeply cyanosed neonate with pulmonary atresia may be dependent on his ductus for survival, and prostaglandins can be administered to keep it open until more definitive treatment is available.

Brettt's PDA was of moderate size and symptomatic with no chance of spontaneous closure. Surgery was therefore undertaken. With the more common situation of a small PDA, surgery can be deferred until 3 years of age. Operative mortality is less than 0.5 per cent compared with a greater than 2 per cent mortality risk throughout life from infective endocarditis. Complications of PDA such as Eisenmenger syndrome are now extremely rare, so the prognosis is excellent.

Coarctation of the Aorta

David, a 14 year old, took himself to the doctor because of increasingly severe frontal headaches. The blood pressure in his left arm was found to be 170/110 mm Hg, and his fundi were normal. His femoral pulses, however, were absent. A cardiologist found that the blood pressure was similar in both arms. He was just able to feel the femoral pulses and measured the lower limb blood pressure with Doppler ultrasound. The systolic pressure was 120 mm Hg.

David's apex beat, which was displaced downwards to the 6th intercostal space, had a forceful impulse. There were no thrills palpable, but a clicking sound was heard in midsystole over the aortic area and this noise was transmitted to the apex. The heart sounds were normal but a continuous murmur was audible over the midthoracic spine (Fig. 4.7).

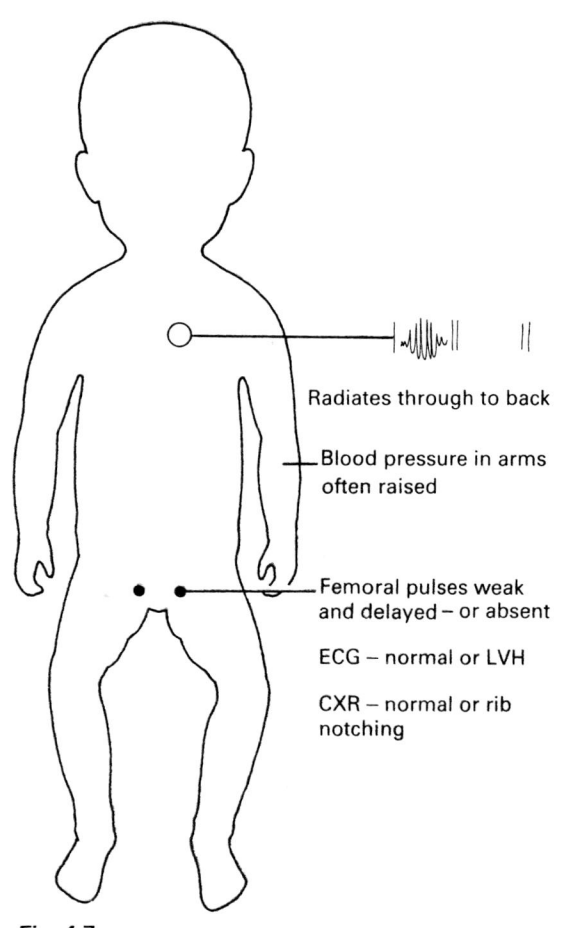

Fig. 4.7
Physical signs of coarctation

- Radiates through to back
- Blood pressure in arms often raised
- Femoral pulses weak and delayed – or absent
- ECG – normal or LVH
- CXR – normal or rib notching

An ECG showed left ventricular hypertrophy and a chest x-ray a large aortic arch but no rib notching. His echocardiogram showed a normal heart except for a bicuspid aortic valve.

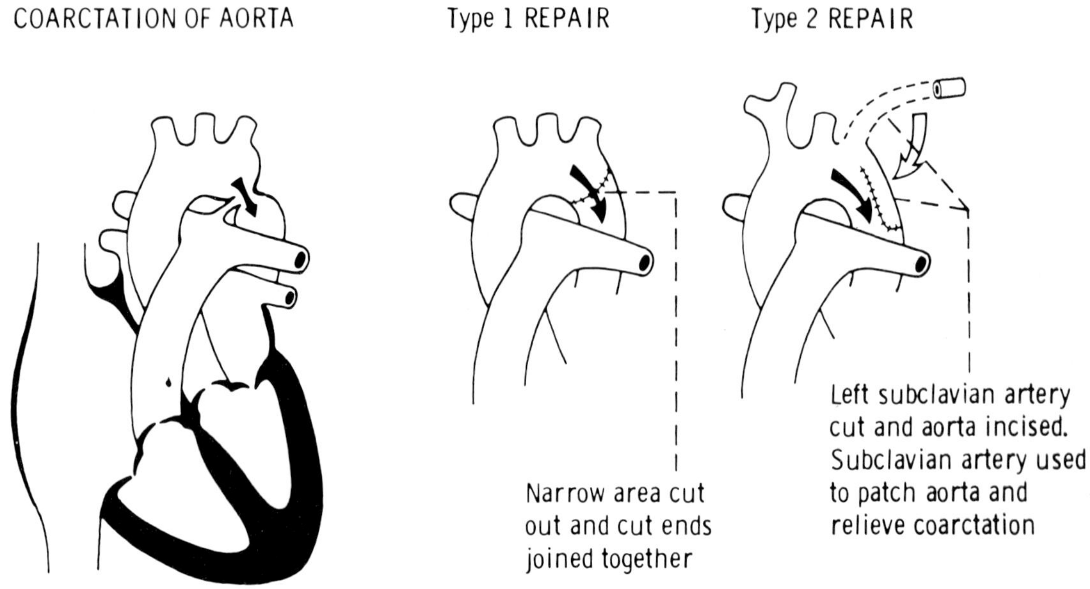

COARCTATION OF AORTA   Type 1 REPAIR   Type 2 REPAIR

Narrow area cut out and cut ends joined together

Left subclavian artery cut and aorta incised. Subclavian artery used to patch aorta and relieve coarctation

Fig. 4.8
Anatomy of coarctation

Comment

Coarctation accounts for 8 per cent of congenital heart disease (Fig. 4.8). Those infants who present in the first few weeks of life with heart failure usually have other associated cardiac anomalies such as a ventricular septal defect or a ductus, and have a high mortality. Children who present after 1 year of age are asymptomatic, the diagnosis being made from absent pulses, murmurs or hypertension. Delay of the femoral pulse compared with the carotid or brachial pulse is a difficult physical sign which is often only found after the diagnosis has already been made!

The Doppler machine is especially useful for the measurement of blood pressure in infants and children. Supine lower limb blood pressure is generally marginally higher than that in the arms but in coarctation of the aorta it is often considerably lower. Hypertension of moderate or severe degree in children is a secondary phenomenon with underlying pathology until proved otherwise although coarctation is not the commonest cause (Table 4.4).

Table 4.4
Causes of hypertension in children

Renal disease (e.g. chronic pyelonephritis)
Coarctation of the aorta
Adrenal disease (e.g. congenital adrenal hyperplasia)
Raised intracranial pressure (e.g. cerebral tumour)
Iatrogenic following fluid overload
Essential hypertension

Most children with moderate or severe hypertension have renal disease.

Bicuspid aortic valves are found in 60 per cent of cases of coarctation, making echocardiography a very helpful investigation. The natural history of coarctation points towards an increasing morbidity and mortality after 20 years of age if untreated (Table 4.5).

Table 4.5
Complications of coarctation of the aorta

Hypertension which persists
Congestive cardiac failure
Infective endocarditis
Subarachnoid haemorrhage (from rupture of an aneurysm)

David had a 5-cm segment of aorta below the origin of the left subclavian artery removed and a Dacron graft inserted to bridge the gap (Fig. 4.9). Postoperatively his femoral pulses returned and his blood pressure fell to normal (105/75 mm Hg). The bicuspid valve may calcify or stenose in middle age, but the main risk to this valve is infective endocarditis. David will always need antibiotic prophylaxis for major dental procedures and surgery likely to lead to bacteraemia. His prognosis is good and no restrictions will be needed.

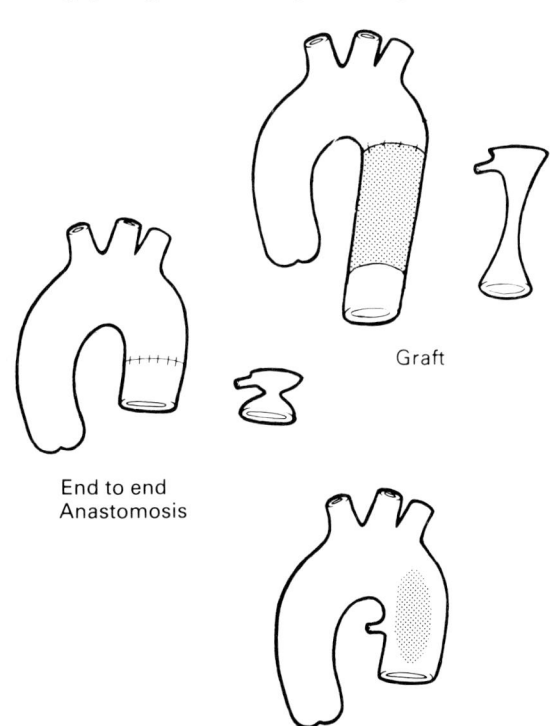

Pulmonary Stenosis

Andrew, a fit 7 year old and a promising footballer, was examined by his family doctor because of a cough. Much to the surprise of the doctor a loud systolic murmur was found, and he was referred for a second opinion.

There was no relevant history and examination showed a pink, tall child who had normal peripheral pulses. A left parasternal heave was just palpable over the precordium, and a systolic thrill was felt at the upper left sternal border when Andrew sat forwards. There was a loud, harsh, ejection systolic murmur heard in the pulmonary area with a quiet, delayed pulmonary second sound.

An echocardiogram excluded other heart disease and showed abnormal valve movements suggestive of pulmonary stenosis. On x-ray the heart was a normal size and shape, with a prominent main pulmonary artery and normal lung fields. The ECG showed right ventricular hypertrophy (Fig. 4.10). These are the features of pulmonary stenosis.

Fig. 4.9
Surgical repair of coarctation

Comment

Pulmonary stenosis is the commonest congenital valve defect, with an incidence of 1 in 1500 children. It can be associated with more complex disease, such as Fallot's tetralogy. Andrew's presentation is typical and since there is no shunting of blood from the pulmonary to the systemic circulation (right to left shunt) cyanosis is absent.

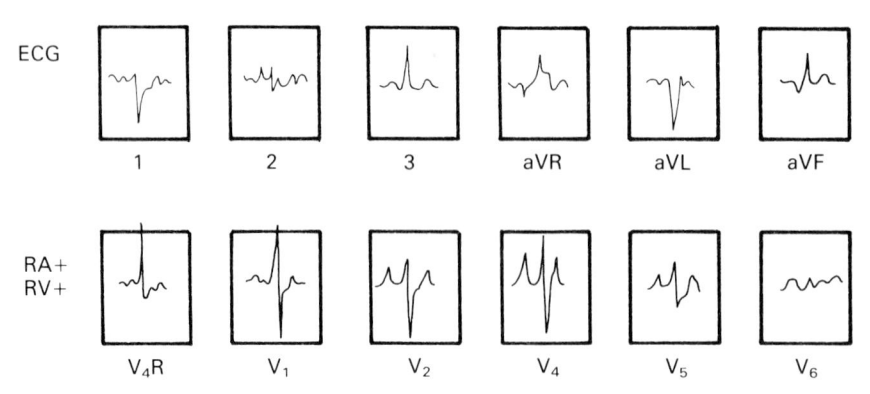

Fig. 4.10
ECG showing right ventricular hypertrophy

When there are symptoms, cyanosis or early heart failure is present, or there is increasing right ventricular hypertrophy on ECG, cardiac catheterization will be indicated. Pressure measurements in the right ventricle and pulmonary artery will help in deciding whether operation is necessary (Fig. 4.11). Generally, if the pressure reaches 75–80 mm Hg in the right ventricle (normal 25 mm Hg), cardiac surgery is indicated because of the risk of damage to the heart muscle which may give rise to heart failure and early death in middle age.

Follow-up is necessary, especially during the adolescent growth spurt as the pressure may rise because growth of the valve orifice fails to keep pace with the increase in stroke volume. As with all congenital heart disease, advice will be given on antibiotic prophylaxis during major dental procedures for prevention of infective endocarditis (Figs. 4.12 and 4.13).

The long-term outlook for mild cases is excellent without treatment. There are insufficient follow-up data on surgically treated cases to give an accurate prognosis on severe cases, but it is hoped that early demise in middle age will be prevented. Andrew can continue with his football as no restrictions on exercise are needed.

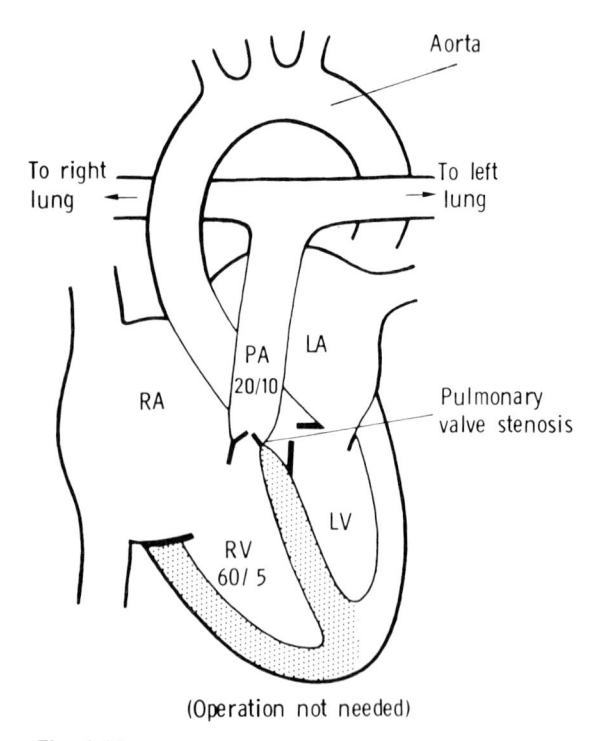

Fig. 4.11
Pressure measurements at cardiac catheterisation in moderate pulmonary stenosis

Ventricular Septal Defect

Fay, a 4-month-old infant whose weight had fallen below the 3rd centile, was admitted to

CARDIOVASCULAR DISEASES

**QUEEN'S MEDICAL CENTRE
NOTTINGHAM**

CHILDREN'S HEART CLINIC

**TEL: NOTTINGHAM 700111
EXT: 3241**

CHILDS NAME: _____

HOSPITAL NO: _____

Fig. 4.12
Antibiotic prophylaxis card

hospital for investigation of failure to thrive. Her father, who gave the history, said she became sweaty and breathless during feeds and that she had only been able to take 55–85 ml (2–3 oz) of milk at each feed during the last few days. There was no relevant perinatal history and the routine examination at 2 days of age had been normal. Fay was the only child of 18-year-old parents.

She was pink in air, had a heart rate of 160 per minute at rest and a respiratory rate of 75 per minute. There was marked intercostal recession and the sternum looked prominent. A systolic thrill was felt to the left of the lower sternal edge and the apex beat was displaced to the anterior axillary line. On auscultation there was a loud pulmonary component of the second heart sound, a pansystolic murmur over the site of the thrill and a suggestion of a diastolic flow murmur at the apex. The liver was enlarged to 5 cm below the costal margin.

These are the features of a ventricular septal defect, or VSD (Fig. 4.14). The ECG showed biventricular hypertrophy. The chest x-ray showed an enlarged heart with pulmonary plethora. Heart failure (Fig. 4.15) was present so the VSD was of moderate to large size. Medical therapy for heart failure was instituted (Table 4.6) and within 48 hours there

TO THE PARENTS

PLEASE SHOW THIS CARD
TO YOUR DENTIST WHEN YOUR
CHILD GOES FOR TREATMENT
MAKE SURE YOUR CHILD
USES A TOOTHBRUSH
PROPERLY, MORNING AND
EVENING

**VISIT YOUR DENTIST
REGULARLY**

TO THE DENTIST

THIS CHILD HAS A CONGENITAL
HEART LESION AND NEEDS ANTI-
BIOTIC PROPHYLAXIS AGAINST
INFECTIVE CARDITIS BEFORE DENTAL
TREATMENT (EXTRACTIONS, FILLINGS
SCALING AND POLISHING)
AMOXYCILLIN (AMOXIL) SHOULD
BE GIVEN IN A SINGLE DOSE ONE
HOUR BEFORE TREATMENT
   10 yrs AND OVER - DOSE 3g
   LESS THAN TEN YRS - DOSE 1 5g
FOR PENICILLIN ALLERGY USE
ERYTHROMICIN 1g ORALLY ONE
HOUR BEFORE TREATMENT
   (HALF DOSE UNDER 10 YRS)

Fig. 4.13
Antibiotic prophylaxis recommendations

50 CLINICAL CASES IN PAEDIATRICS

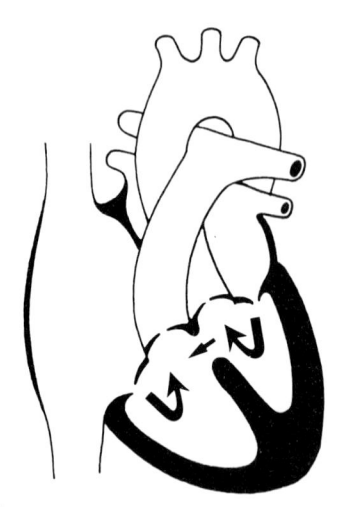

Fig. 4.14
Anatomy of VSD

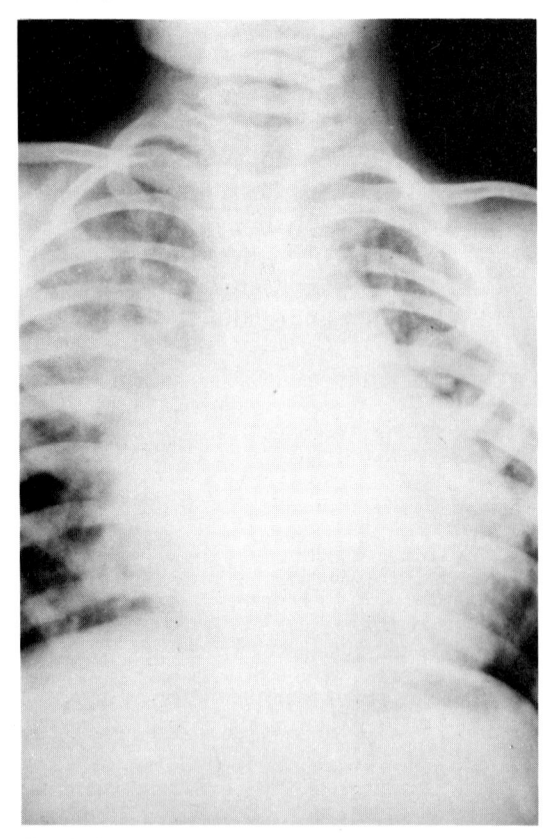

Fig. 4.15
Chest x-ray in child with large VSD

Table 4.6
Medical treatment of heart failure in infancy

Nurse sitting up
Nasogastric feeding
Diuretics (frusemide, spironolactone)
Digoxin
Oxygen if there is pulmonary oedema or central cyanosis

was a dramatic improvement in Fay's general condition.

A cardiac catheter study confirmed the presence of a moderately large VSD, with a 3 to 1 shunt so that there was three times as much blood flow to the lungs as to the systemic circulation. Pressure measurements showed only moderate elevation in the main pulmonary artery, which returned to normal when 100% oxygen was given (Fig. 4.16). This

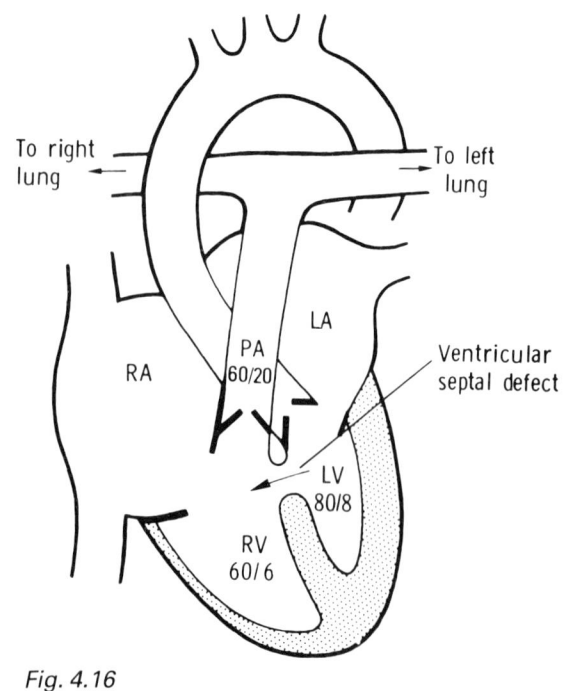

Fig. 4.16
Diagram of moderate VSD, with pressures found during cardiac catheterization

meant that the pulmonary hypertension was reversible and that there was no irreversible damage to the small blood vessels of the lungs.

Comment

VSDs account for a quarter of all congenital heart disease. Fortunately, most lesions are small and asymptomatic, and only require occasional follow-up. All types require antibiotic prophylaxis to prevent infective endocarditis. The natural history of the disease suggests that most VSDs will close spontaneously (Fig. 4.17), so catheter studies are indicated only for those at high risk of complications.

Infants who present in heart failure which responds to treatment have a hole that tends to stay the same size, and so it becomes relatively smaller as the child grows. With intractable heart failure and in situations where the catheter study suggests a high risk of future problems, a one-stage total correction will be undertaken.

Fay's heart failure lessened over the next few months so anti-failure treatment was stopped, and she thrived satisfactorily. The murmur disappeared between her 18- and 24-month visit, indicating that spontaneous closure had taken place.

Fallot's Tetralogy

Stuart was 3 years old and had presented at 3 months of age with dusky colouration of his lips when crying and feeding. He was pink at rest and on examination was found to have a single pulmonary second heart sound and an ejection systolic murmur over the left upper chest. During the next 15 months he became centrally cyanosed at rest and finger clubbing developed. A chest x-ray showed a boot-shaped heart with a prominent right ventricle (Fig. 4.18) and the ECG revealed right axis deviation and right ventricular hypertrophy.

Stuart was seen by a paediatric cardiologist, who performed an echocardiogram which showed a hypertrophied right ventricle with a small outlet, an aorta overriding both ventricles and a large ventricular septal defect. A cardiac catheter study using pressure measurements and cineradiography confirmed the diagnosis of Fallot's tetralogy (Fig. 4.19).

Stuart had become increasingly disabled during the few months after he was seen, with a markedly reduced exercise tolerance, and he was noted to be more polycythaemic. When upset he had hypercyanotic episodes, his mother commenting that his lips became black and that he became floppy and lifeless for several minutes. When tired, he tended to squat down on the floor. An urgent referral for total corrective surgery under cardiopulmonary bypass was arranged.

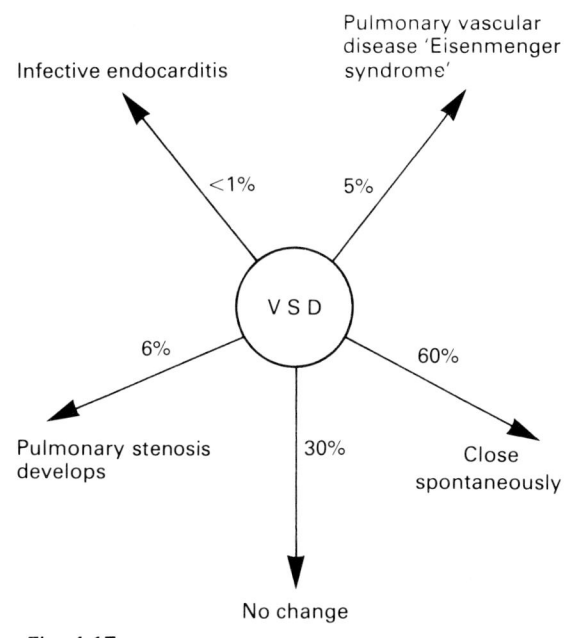

Fig. 4.17
Natural history of VSD

- Infective endocarditis <1%
- Pulmonary vascular disease 'Eisenmenger syndrome' 5%
- Close spontaneously 60%
- No change 30%
- Pulmonary stenosis develops 6%

52 CLINICAL CASES IN PAEDIATRICS

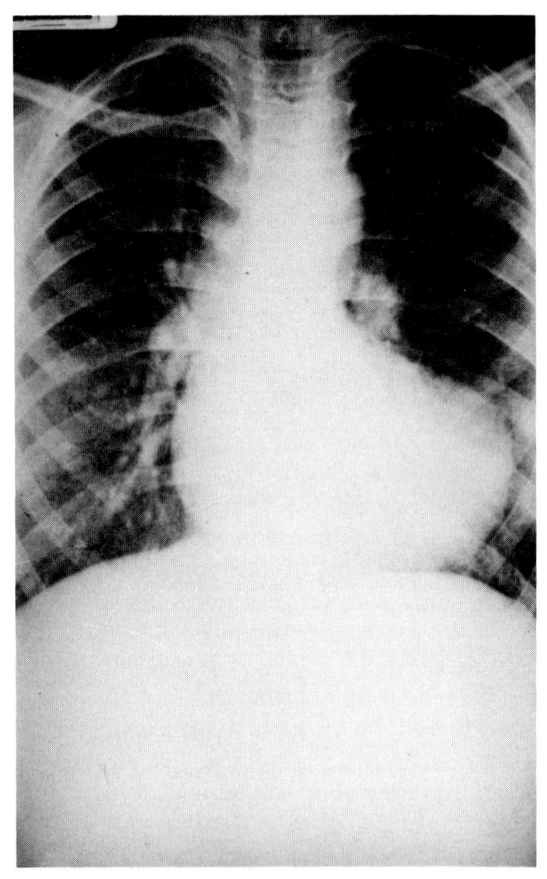

Fig. 4.18
Chest x-ray of child with Fallot's tetralogy

Comment

Corrective surgery for Fallot's tetralogy has a 10 per cent mortality, but, untreated, 90 per cent of patients will die before the age of 25, with a poor quality of life prior to death. Sometimes infants can present in the first few weeks of life with cyanosis. Inevitably they have more severe obstruction to blood flow out of the right ventricle. A palliative shunt operation such as a Blalock procedure (subclavian artery to pulmonary artery anastomosis) will be needed as an initial procedure to increase blood flow to the lungs.

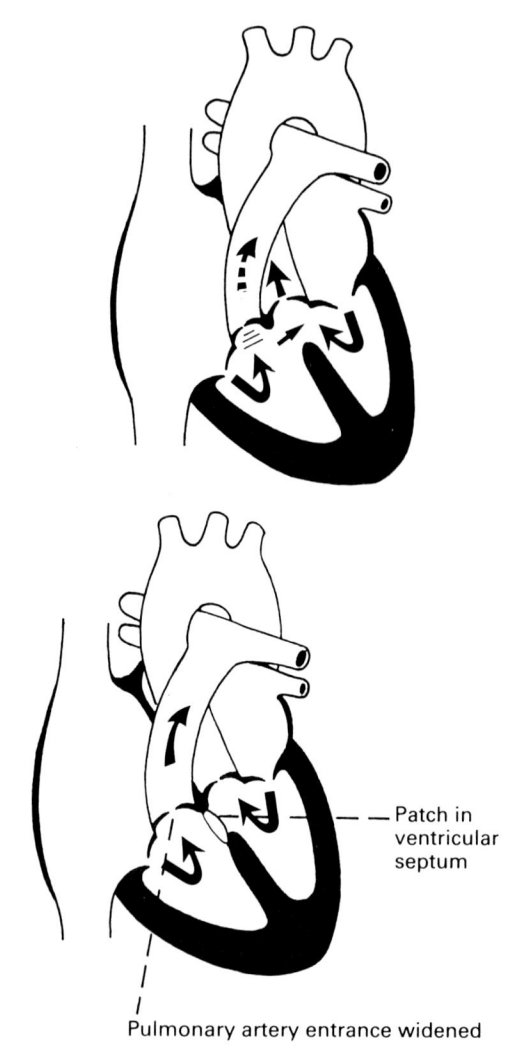

Fig. 4.19
Anatomy of Fallot's tetralogy, with method of surgical repair

Total corrective surgery has occasionally been performed in the first few months of life, but is generally reserved for children over the age of a year. The long-term outlook following total correction appears excellent and the majority of successful operations render the child asymptomatic and able to return to a normal life.

5 Gastroenterology

Infectious Hepatitis

Amanda, aged 10 years, had been unwell for several days with poor appetite, nausea and vague abdominal pains. Her two older brothers and her parents were well, although Amanda's mother suffered from intermittent acute anxiety. Her father was company director of a textile firm which had just called in the Official Receiver. There was no diarrhoea, fever or history of contact with infectious disease.

The family doctor was summoned for the second time in three days by Amanda's upset mother, who said she felt Amanda needed to be in hospital. He examined Amanda again and found a slightly tender liver, and a spleen tip that was just palpable. There was no jaundice, but a urine test with a Multistix showed a positive test for bilirubin. Feeling that viral hepatitis was probable, he had a long discussion with both parents to reassure them, explaining that there was no specific treatment and Amanda could get up out of bed when she felt better. A blood sample was taken for liver function tests and to see if hepatitis B surface antigen was present (Table 5.1). These results showed a slight elevation in bilirubin and very high transaminase levels indicating liver damage. In the absence of drug ingestion and with no evidence of hepatitis B infection, viral hepatitis A was very likely.

Comment

A number of drugs are capable of producing liver damage (Table 5.2), and this cause should be excluded in any patient with liver disease. There are also a wide variety of infectious agents causing hepatitis (Table 5.3), and there are specific tests available for diagnosing most (including hepatitis A virus infection). These are not routine tests and will hardly contribute to the management of a child with hepatitis being treated at home. It is important to exclude hepatitis B infection, as this has a much worse prognosis and specific mea-

Table 5.1

Amanda's blood results (normal range in parentheses)

Bilirubin	27 μmol/l (5–17)
Asparate transaminase	660 IU/l (5–15)
Alanine transaminase	884 IU/l (5–30)
Alkaline phosphatase	210 IU/l (80–180)
Hepatitis B surface antigen	negative

Table 5.2

Some drugs which are capable of causing liver damage

Sodium valproate
Paracetamol (overdose)
Halothane
Chlorpromazine
Rifampicin

sures will need to be taken to protect the family (see below).

Hepatitis A virus infection is present throughout the world, and is common in children. Viral transmission occurs in situations of overcrowding and poor sanitation, as transmission is by the faeco-oral route. The frequency of anicteric hepatitis, which can be impossible to diagnose, varies with age. In the preschool age the ratio of anicteric to icteric children is 10:1, whereas for teenagers and young adults it is 1:1. The disease is notifiable in the UK.

Table 5.3

Infectious agents causing jaundice

Viruses:
    Hepatitis A, B, and non-A non-B
    Glandular fever (Epstein–Barr virus)
    Cytomegalovirus
    Yellow fever
    Congenital rubella and herpes viruses
Bacteria:
    Brucellosis
    Leptospirosis
Parasites:
    Amoebic hepatitis
    Malaria

Prophylaxis for hepatitis A is effective within two weeks of exposure, and may be given to contacts or to children travelling to the tropics. Pooled gammaglobulin gives passive protection for up to seven months. Specific hyperimmune hepatitis B globulin is now available for prophylaxis against hepatitis B. Active immunization with attenuated hepatitis B vaccine is also now available. The prognosis is excellent for hepatitis A. There is no risk of a chronic carrier state and a single infection produces life-long immunity.

Gastroenteritis

Leon, an only child who was 4 months old, was taken to his family doctor after a two-day illness, which his mother described as 'a bit of a tummy upset'. The health visitor had been concerned about Leon's recent weight gain, as he had a birth weight of 2.8 kg and now weighed 4 kg. Numerous home visits had been unsuccessful because of failure to keep appointments—there was nobody at home. There had also been concern about the amount of support the mother was getting from her husband, who seemed to spend most of his time (and unemployment benefit) in the pub.

It was difficult to elicit an accurate history but it appeared that the main problem was diarrhoea up to 15 times each day for the last 48 hours and loss of interest in his bottle feeds. In spite of the mother's apparent lack of concern, the infant looked ill, with a tachycardia of 180 per minute and a poor volume pulse. He had both sunken eyes and fontanelle (Fig. 5.1) and a scaphoid abdomen with decreased skin turgor so that the skin did not spring back in place when pinched (Fig. 5.2). The extremities were cool. These are the features of 10 per cent dehydration (Table 5.4).

Leon had acute gastroenteritis (Fig. 5.3) and was urgently admitted to hospital for resuscitation with intravenous plasma. This dramatically improved his general condition. Stool cultures, blood gases and biochemistry specimens were sent off to the laboratory.

Comment

The disease is caused by a bowel infection, the commonest pathogen in the UK being rotavirus. Five per cent of all children will develop gastroenteritis during their first year of life, but the majority can be managed at

GASTROENTEROLOGY 55

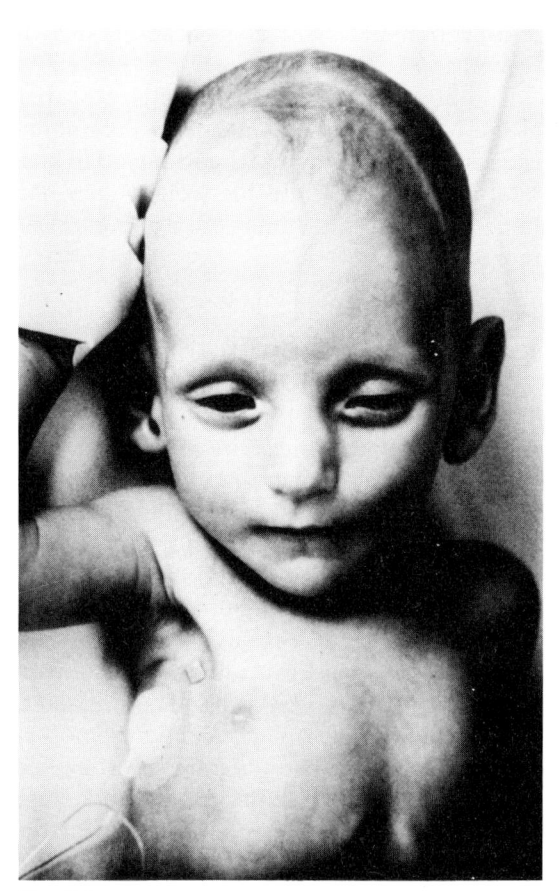

Fig. 5.1
Sunken fontanelle in severe dehydration

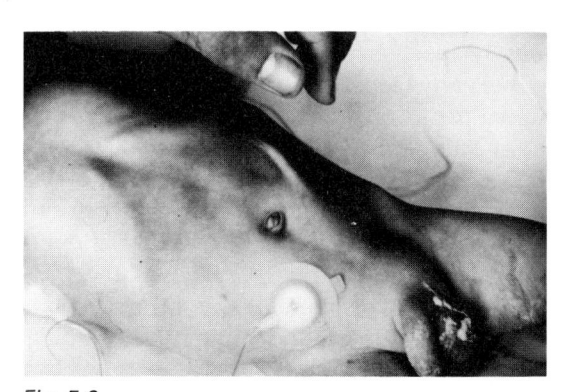

Fig. 5.2
Decreased skin turgor in severe dehydration

Table 5.4
Clinical assessment of dehydration

Clinical features	Degree of dehydration
Undetectable	<3%
Loss of skin turgor, dry mouth	3–5%
Depressed fontanelle, slightly sunken eyes, good peripheral circulation	5%
Tachycardia, hypotension, peripheral shutdown, grossly sunken eyes	10%
Moribund	12%

ACUTE GASTROENTERITIS

- Fontanelle depressed
- Sunken eyes
- Dry mouth
- Deep acidotic breathing
- Scaphoid abdomen bowel sounds++
- Rapid thready pulse

Diarrhoea ± vomiting

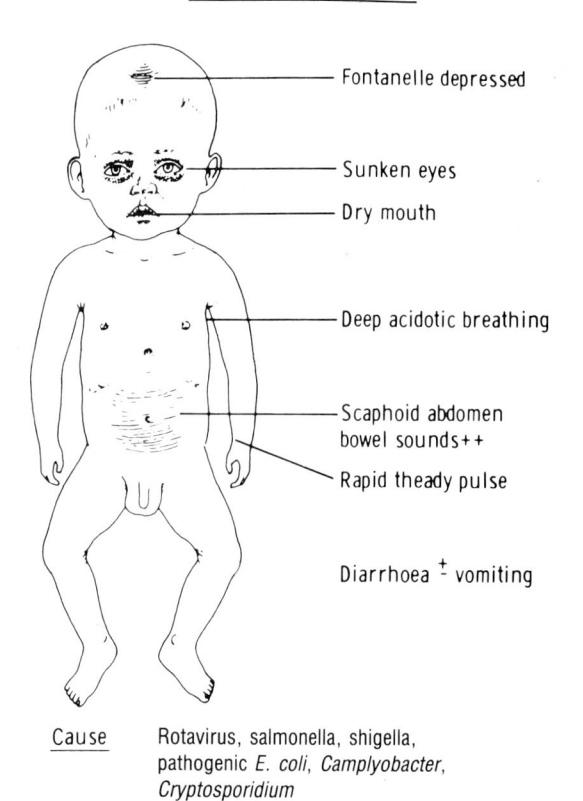

Cause — Rotavirus, salmonella, shigella, pathogenic *E. coli*, *Camplyobacter*, *Cryptosporidium*

Fig. 5.3
Physical signs of severe gastroenteritis

home. Hospital admission is required for ill children or more often when there are co-existent social problems. Breast feeding protects against gastroenteritis. The peak incidence is at between 9 months and 2 years, and there are about ten million deaths annually in infants in Asia, Africa and Latin America.

In mild cases, small frequent milk feeds are needed, but in more severe cases only clear fluids are given orally. A sugar such as glucose should be present, being important not only as an energy source but also as a 'driving force' for the absorption of fluids and electrolytes. Small quantities of fluid are given at frequent intervals, but if vomiting continues or there are signs of shock, intravenous fluid will be needed.

The quantity of oral or intravenous fluid is calculated by the estimation of maintenance requirements and adding the fluid deficit due to dehydration. There are a number of oral solutions suitable for rehydration in mild to moderate cases, made by adding sachets of powder to boiled water. Rice water is sometimes used in the tropics. If intravenous therapy is used, half physiological (normal) saline with 2.5% dextrose is given until the electrolyte results are available. The serum sodium determines the type of fluid to follow on and the time taken to correct the deficit. If the level is normal or low, correction is carried out over 24 hours. If there is hypernatraemia, rehydration is given over 48 hours in an attempt to prevent neurological complications such as convulsions.

Complications of gastroenteritis can arise (Table 5.5), and it is still one of the commoner causes of death in infants. Leon stayed in hospital for a month until his weight gain had improved and the home environment was more stable.

Recurrent Abdominal Pain

Scott was an 8-year-old boy who had recently referred to a paediatrician by his general practitioner because of recurrent abdominal pain.

He was born at full term, after a normal pregnancy and delivery, weighing 2.80 kg and had no neonatal illnesses. His abdominal pain had been occurring in bouts for about 12 months, and he would have episodes every four weeks lasting for up to a day. The pain was central and lower abdominal, and associated with vomiting on occasions. His mother said that when he had the pain, Scott looked pale and ill, with large pupils and dark rings around his eyes. During an episode of the pain he would lie down on his bed and not eat anything until the pain had gone, missing school for a couple of days. She described him as a quiet, sensitive boy who took things to heart easily. She herself was a smallish woman who suffered from frequent migrainous headaches which began when she was in her early teens. She, too, had bouts of abdominal pain as a child, and during one episode a normal appendix was removed. Scott's father was a travelling salesman who was away from home for most of the week. He had two siblings, a 3-year-old sister and a 6-year-old brother Craig. Craig was the complete opposite of Scott. He was a big boy, good looking, extrovert and aggressive, popular with family and friends alike.

On examination, Scott was a small boy, with a height and weight on the 3rd percentile

Table 5.5

Complications of gastroenteritis

Early	Dehydration
	Acute renal failure
	Cerebral or renal vein thrombosis
	Electrolyte disturbance with convulsions
Late	Persisting food intolerance, especially to lactose

GASTROENTEROLOGY 57

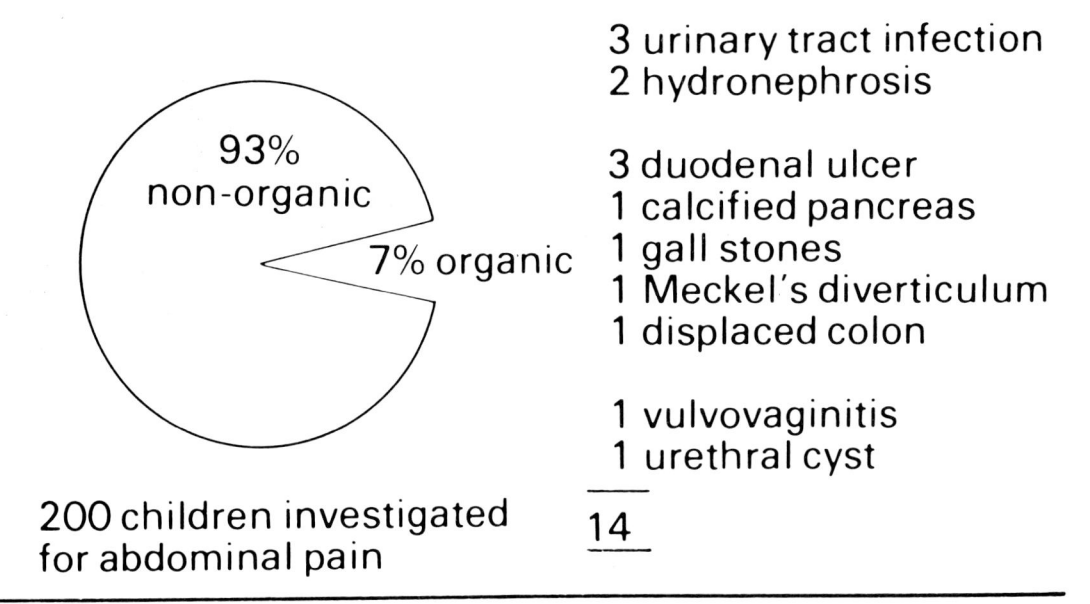

```
                           3 urinary tract infection
                           2 hydronephrosis
      93%
   non-organic             3 duodenal ulcer
                           1 calcified pancreas
       7% organic          1 gall stones
                           1 Meckel's diverticulum
                           1 displaced colon

                           1 vulvovaginitis
                           1 urethral cyst
  200 children investigated
  for abdominal pain       14
```

Fig. 5.4
Aetiology of abdominal pain (*after Apley*)

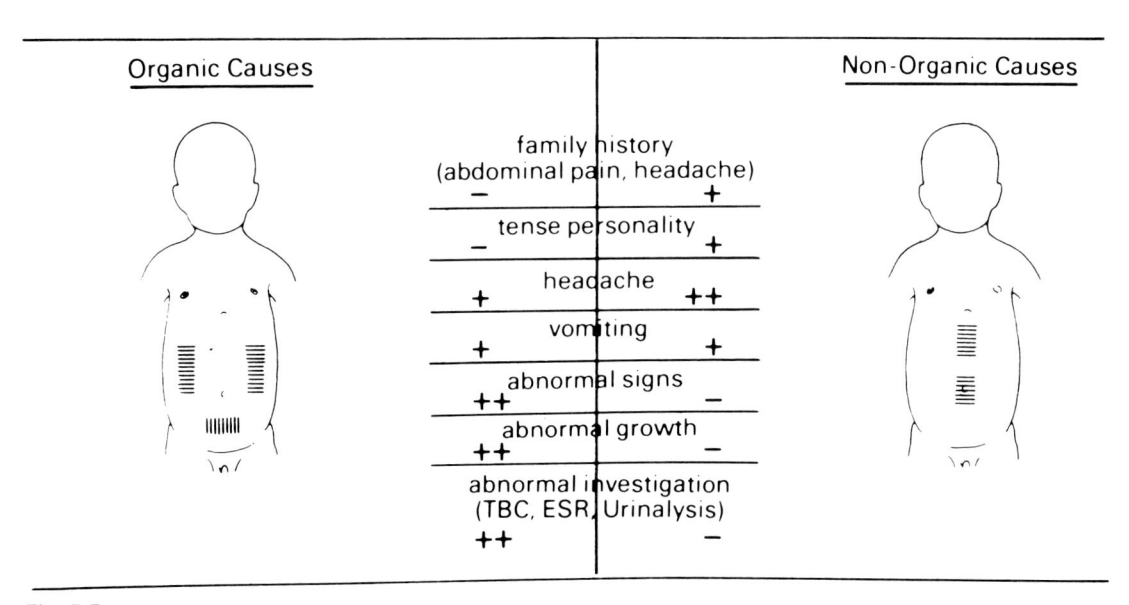

Organic Causes			Non-Organic Causes
	family history (abdominal pain, headache)		
	−	+	
	tense personality		
	−	+	
	headache		
	+	++	
	vomiting		
	+	+	
	abnormal signs		
	++	−	
	abnormal growth		
	++	−	
	abnormal investigation (TBC, ESR, Urinalysis)		
	++	−	

Fig. 5.5
Features suggestive of organic abdominal pain (*From Hull D & Johnston DI (1981)* Essential Paediatrics. *Churchill Livingstone, Edinburgh, by courtesy of the publishers*)

for his age. There were no abnormal physical findings. A urine culture showed no infection.

Comment

Scott has the typical features of recurrent abdominal pain due to non-organic causes and has many of the personality traits described in such children. Dr John Apley studied 200 children with recurrent abdominal pain and found that only 7 per cent had an organic cause (Fig. 5.4). Urine culture is mandatory in all such children, and barium studies or endoscopy will be indicated in the few children who have upper abdominal pain and tenderness, as peptic ulceration is a commonly missed diagnosis (Fig. 5.5).

Recurrent abdominal pain affects 10 per cent of school children and is often associated with headaches and vomiting. The paediatrician spent some time with Scott and his mother explaining that although psychogenic in nature, the pain is real to Scott. It was suggested that the family try to play down his symptoms as much as possible, with the minimum of fuss. Scott appeared to be overshadowed by his younger brother, and his mother was made aware of this as a stress-inducing mechanism.

The prognosis is not as good as might be expected. Many 'little bellyachers' grow up to be 'big bellyachers' or develop migraine.

Herpes Stomatitis

Sally, a 1 year old, was on holiday with her parents and became unwell, fretful and irritable. She was not willing to eat or drink and the next morning her mouth became extremely sore. After she had not drunk for 24 hours her parents took her to the local accident and emergency department.

Sally was an only child of unmarried parents. Her mother, who was now six months pregnant, was 18 years old, and her father was a 19-year-old car mechanic. The social services had previously been involved with the family because of worries about care of the child and the possibility of neglect. Sally's father gave little support to the family. Nevertheless the situation appeared stable most of the time, with full involvement of community services.

When Sally was seen in the accident and emergency department she was an ill, pyrexial child with a temperature of 40°C and mild dehydration. Just inside her mouth were yellow vesicles on a red inflamed base; these lesions were ulcerated over the tongue, palate, gums and pharynx. The cervical lymph nodes were tender and moderately enlarged and the spleen tip was just palpable, Admission to hospital took place and the dehydration corrected with oral fluids. No specific treatment was given but she improved over the next three days and she was discharged home after a week.

Comment

Nearly all cases of acute gingivostomatitis in young children are due to primary herpes simplex virus infection. Laboratory confirmation by virus isolation from the lesions, or rising antibody titres, is unnecessary as the diagnosis is clinically obvious. Herpangina caused by Coxsackie A virus produces similar lesions on the soft palate and anterior fauces but there is no gingivitis. The majority of primary herpes infections are asymptomatic, but in 1 per cent of cases a wide variety of unpleasant and occasionally lethal manifestations are seen (Table 5.6). The ubiquity of this virus is generally not appreciated because, in contrast with herpes zoster, symptoms are rarely present (Fig. 5.6). Approximately 80 per cent of adults are carriers of the herpes simplex

Table 5.6
Primary infections with herpes simplex virus

Subclinical (99%)
Clinical illness (1%)   Gingivostomatitis
                        Vulvovaginitis
                        Keratoconjunctivitis
                        Encephalitis
                        Eczema herpeticum

Table 5.7
Reactivation of herpes simplex virus

Recurrent cold sores around the lips
Genital herpes
Dendritic corneal ulcers

tion in an immunocompromised child (e.g. with leukaemia) may be devastating. Acyclovir, an antiviral agent which is especially active against the herpes group of viruses, can be given locally or parenterally to reduce morbidity and mortality.

As with most disease in children, social factors affect both the time of presentation and the ability of the family to cope. In view of the initial delay in seeking medical attention, Sally was kept in hospital until she was back on a normal diet. The parents were reassured that a similar infection would not arise again.

Hirschsprung's Disease

Mandy was seen for her routine check at 6 weeks of age at her local child health clinic.

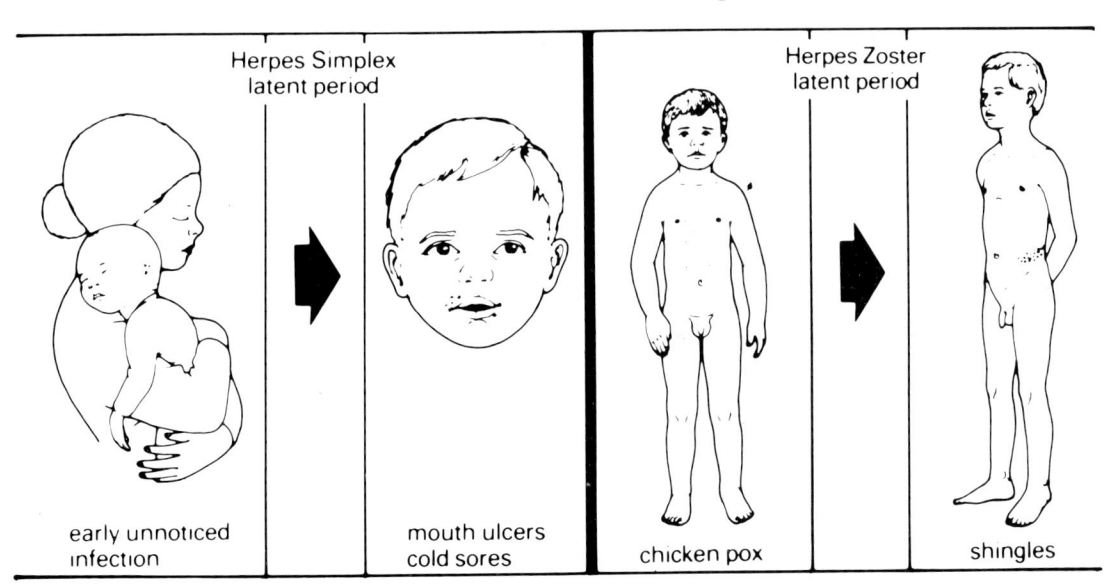

Herpes Simplex latent period		Herpes Zoster latent period	
early unnoticed infection	mouth ulcers cold sores	chicken pox	shingles

Fig. 5.6
Contrasting features of herpes simplex and zoster infections (*From Milner AD & Hull D (1984)* Hospital Paediatrics. *Churchill Livingstone, Edinburgh, by courtesy of the publishers*)

virus, and reactivation symptoms may occur (Table 5.7).

Specific antiviral treatment is not given to the normal child with herpes stomatitis as the illness is self limiting. However, such an infec-

The health visitor was concerned about the combination of constipation in association with a weight gain of only 500 g since birth. The baby had a birth weight of 3.30 kg and was born following a normal pregnancy, labour and delivery. When examined, Mandy looked unwell, had muscle wasting and obvious abdominal distension. The rectum was free of faeces and felt small.

The clinic doctor felt that an organic cause for the distension and constipation was likely so he sent Mandy for a second opinion the following week. The paediatrician confirmed the physical signs and arranged hospital admission for further investigation and treatment. The following day a barium enema showed a dilated large bowel with a sudden change of calibre to a small constricted segment (Fig. 5.7). This appearance was thought to be typical of Hirschsprung's disease and Mandy was transferred to a nearby paediatric surgical unit for treatment.

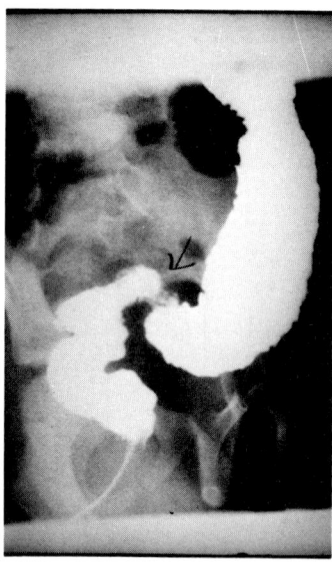

Fig. 5.7
Barium enema in Hirschsprung's disease

Comment

In 1887 Hirschsprung described the condition as a lethal disease of infancy characterized by intractable constipation, gross dilatation of the colon and an empty rectum. The incidence is approximately 1 in 10 000 and 85 per cent of cases present in the first month of life, often as delay in passage of meconium beyond 24 hours after birth.

The condition arises as a result of failure of migration of ganglion cells to the submucosa and myenteric plexuses of the bowel (Fig. 5.8). The rectosigmoid colon is most commonly involved although there can be involvement of the proximal colon (Fig. 5.9). This aganglionic segment is narrow and produces inadequate peristalsis, leading to bowel obstruction with a secondary distension of bowel proximal to this obstruction.

Diagnosis is made by barium enema in most cases, confirmed by rectal biopsy which reveals no ganglion cells. Abnormal function of the internal anal sphincter can be confirmed by anorectal manometry when there is diagnostic difficulty, especially if a very short segment of gut is involved. Treatment of Hirschsprung's disease is surgical, preferably before gross failure to thrive and distension take place. It is best performed by a surgeon familiar with these difficult cases. The principles of treatment involve immediate relief of obstruction, followed by excision of the aganglionic segment with anastomosis of normal bowel to the anal canal (Fig. 5.10).

Neonatal mortality is still around 20 per cent, largely due to the complications of surgery and necrotizing enterocolitis, the incidence of which is related to the degree of bowel obstruction. Most children are continent following surgery, but a small minority will fail to achieve this and will need a permanent colostomy.

Pyloric Stenosis

Nolan, a 3-week-old baby of West Indian parents, was seen because of persistent vomiting after feeds for five days. He had been well up until this time and had been gaining

GASTROENTEROLOGY 61

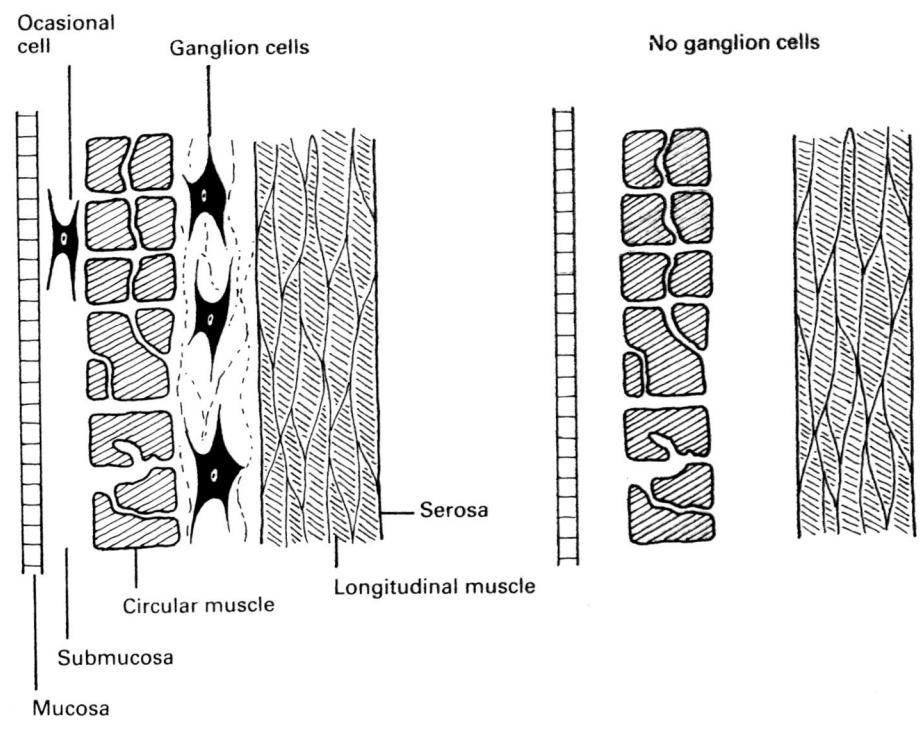

Fig. 5.8
Histology of Hirschsprung's disease

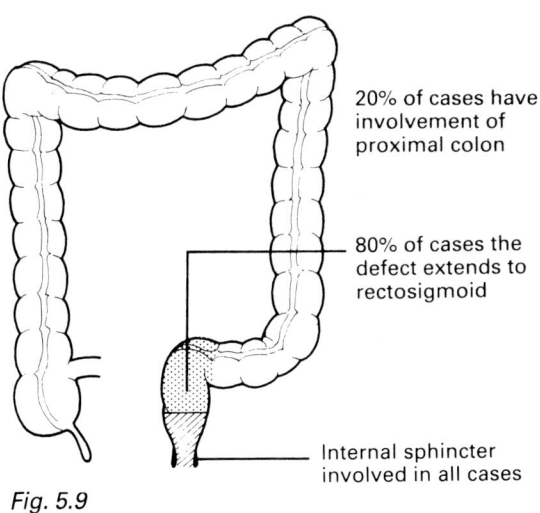

Fig. 5.9
Extent of aganglionic area in Hirschsprung's disease

Fig. 5.10
Operative management of Hirschsprung's disease

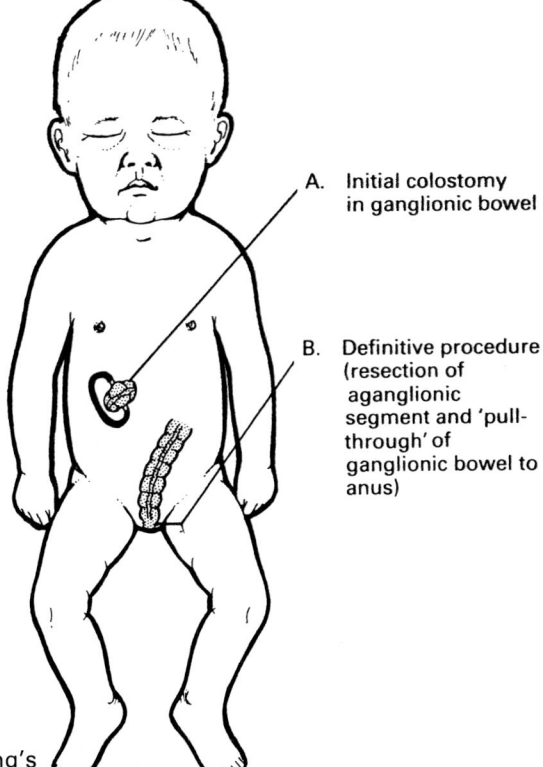

62 CLINICAL CASES IN PAEDIATRICS

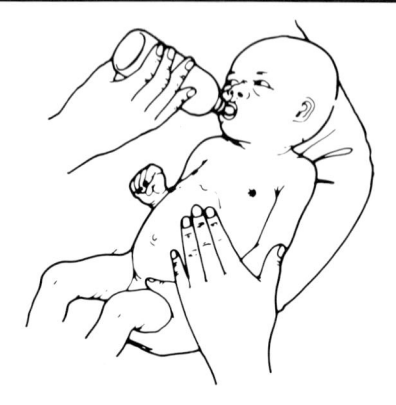

- gently massage

- tumour often felt immediately prior to vomit

- size of tumour varies; hard small ones difficult to palpate

Fig. 5.11
Test feed for pyloric stenosis (*From Milner AD & Hull D (1984)* Hospital Paediatrics. *Churchill Livingstone, Edinburgh, by courtesy of the publishers*)

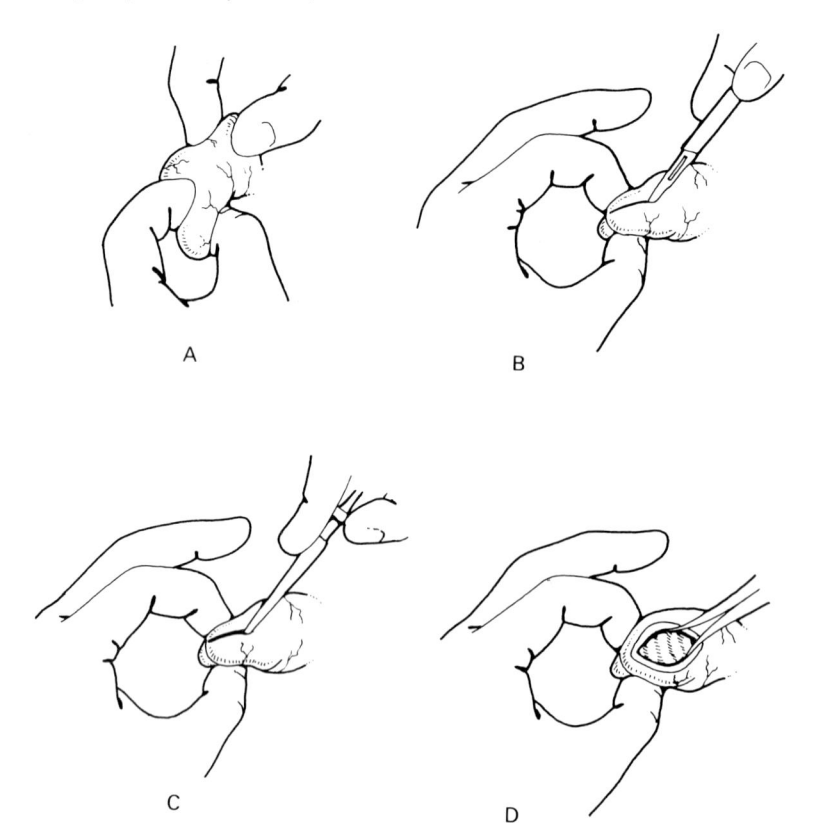

Fig. 5.12
Ramstedt's procedure

weight normally. His brother, a 3 year old, was a fit young lad who had had no vomiting as an infant. On further enquiry there was a suggestion that the vomiting was projectile in nature but no blood or bile had been seen in it. It certainly seemed to be related to feeds.

In view of the symptoms a test feed was carried out (Fig. 5.11), revealing visible gastric peristalsis. A palpable pyloric swelling was present in the right upper quadrant of the baby's abdomen. The tumour felt the size of an olive and moved under the examiner's fingers. The houseman sent off some blood for urea and electrolyte analysis, and was surprised when all the results, including a chloride level, were normal.

The surgeon appeared a few hours later to repeat the test feed to confirm the physical signs. They arranged for an operating theatre and performed a pyloromyotomy (Ramstedt's procedure) under general anaesthetic that afternoon (Fig. 5.12). The operation was uneventful and feeding was recommenced six hours postoperatively. The baby was home three days later.

Comment

The incidence of pyloric stenosis is 3 per 1000 in Great Britain in Caucasians but is less common in Negro or Asian babies. There is a 4:1 male predominance and a familial incidence which suggests that genetic factors are involved. The pylorus is hypertrophied and so gastric emptying is obstructed (Fig. 5.13), which leads to dilatation of the stomach and excessive peristalsis. The vomitus is free of bile as the level of bowel obstruction is above the ampulla of Vater. When there are diagnostic difficulties and typical physical signs are absent, barium studies will enable a diagnosis to be made. Electrolyte disturbances occur because of the loss of water, acid and potassium with vomiting, resulting in hypokalae-

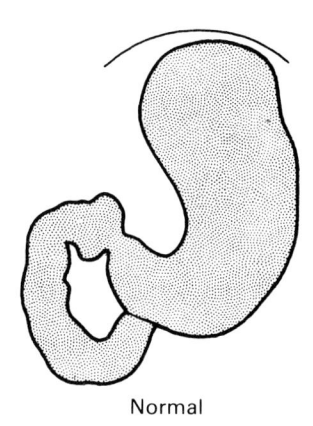

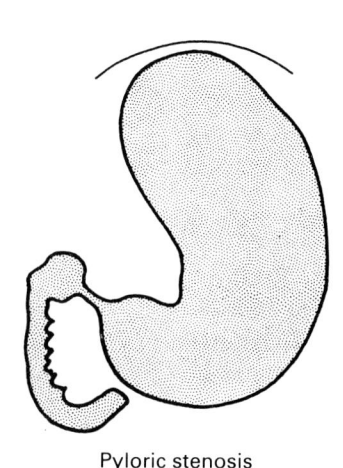

Fig. 5.13
Radiological appearance of pyloric stenosis

Table 5.8

Fluid and electrolyte disturbance in pyloric stenosis

Urea	↑	because of dehydration and prerenal failure
Chloride	↓	because of loss of chloride in vomit
Potassium	↓	because of loss of chloride in vomit
Bicarbonate	↑	Metabolic alkalosis because of loss of acid in vomit and hypokalaemia

mic alkalosis and dehydration (Table 5.8). When the history is short, the urea and electrolytes may be normal.

Operation is never urgent. When there is severe dehydration, fluid and electrolyte losses can be replaced over 48 hours with intravenous dextrose/saline and potassium. Postoperative complications sometimes seen are incomplete myotomy resulting in continuing obstruction and wound dehiscence which is secondary to preoperative malnutrition. Survival should be near 100 per cent and there are few if any long-term complications.

Gastro-oesophageal Reflux

Lisa, a 10-week-old baby, presented with a history of frequent vomiting since birth. Her mother said that she was sick as often as 10–20 times a day, following and between feeds.

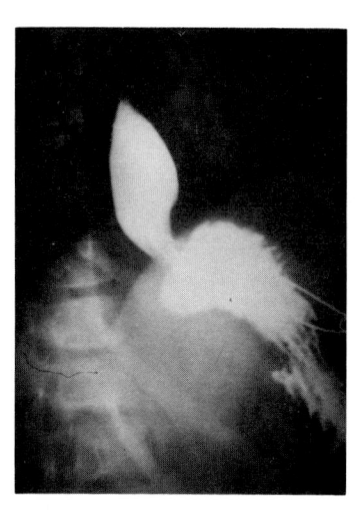

Fig. 5.14
X-ray of sliding hiatus hernia

Small amounts of curdled milk were brought up each time she was sick which made a mess of her clothes, her mother and their house! Lisa herself seemed unconcerned although her weight gain was rather slow. On examination there were no abnormal physical signs and a test feed excluded a diagnosis of pyloric stenosis. In view of the symptoms a barium swallow was carried out which showed a sliding hiatus hernia, part of the stomach lying above the diaphragm (Fig. 5.14). The remainder of the swallow showed no sign of an oesophageal stricture and no pyloric stenosis.

The parents were asked to prop Lisa up at a 45-degree angle in the prone position and the feeds were thickened with a carob powder preparation. A review two weeks later showed that most of the symptoms had subsided and her weight gain had improved. By 7 months of age there were no further symptoms and treatment was discontinued.

Comment

The presenting complaint of reflux is persistent vomiting, usually beginning in the first six weeks of life. Occasionally the vomitus will contain blood or mucus. If the vomiting is severe, a barium swallow is indicated to see if there is a sliding hiatus hernia. This results in gastro-oesophageal reflux due to the absence of lower oesophageal sphincter control. In some cases there may be inflammation of the oesophageal mucosa (reflux oesophagitis) and this occasionally leads to stricture formation. Other varieties of hiatus hernia in infants are uncommon but occasionally the whole stomach may herniate through the diaphragm (Fig. 5.15).

Most infants with reflux have vomiting which tends to subside spontaneously over a few months. More severely affected infants are treated by thickening their milk feeds with an inert powder such as carob powder preparation. Nursing them in the prone position on a slope and the use of antacids also help.

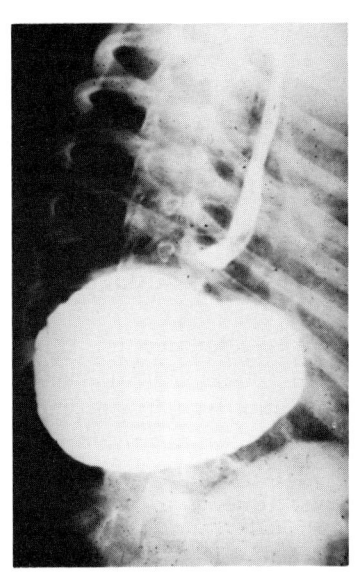

Fig. 5.15
X-ray showing massive hiatus hernia

If there are persistent symptoms after 1 year of age with complications, a laparotomy to perform a fundoplication of the stomach may be indicated. Fortunately the vast majority of infants respond to simple measures and the outlook for this common condition is excellent.

Chronic Constipation

Richard, a 6 year old, had been followed up in the outpatient clinic for nearly two years with constipation that was accompanied by soiling (Table 5.9). He had been seen by a variety of doctors, each of whom prescribed his favourite laxative. Richard's mother had boosted the fibre content of his diet, as well as adding prunes and figs, but to no avail. The school were finding this problem difficult to deal with and had asked the parents if they needed to seek another medical opinion.

In view of the pressure from the parents, a more active management programme was initiated with a ten-day hospital admission during the school holidays. When he was admitted, he had abdominal distension with numerous 'hard rocks' palpable abdominally in addition to a loaded rectum. On the ward, full doses of laxatives were given (Table 5.10) and a daily saline enema. By ten days the faecal masses had disappeared and he was discharged home on laxatives to establish a normal bowel habit. Soiling recommenced several weeks later in spite of the measures, so admission as a day case was undertaken for an anal dilatation under general anaesthe-

Table 5.9
Definitions in constipation

Constipation	Difficulty or delay in the passage of stools
Soiling	Frequent passage of loose or semisolid stools in pants
Encopresis	Passage of a normal stool in an abnormal place

Table 5.10
Laxatives for children

Bulk increasers (holding water within the bowel)	Faecal softeners	Bowel stimulants
High fibre diet Lactulose	Dioctyl sodium sulphosuccinate Liquid paraffin	Senna Bisacodyl Milk of magnesia

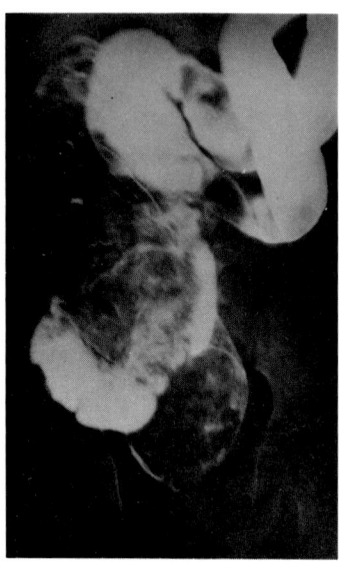

Fig. 5.16
Barium enema showing megacolon

tic. Outpatient investigations prior to this showed a dilated distal colon and rectum on barium enema (Fig. 5.16) and no suggestion of Hirschsprung's disease on anorectal manometry. Richard's soiling ceased after discharge, although laxatives were needed most of the time for the next two years.

Comment

Acute constipation can be triggered by a variety of factors such as fever, dehydration or anorexia. It is a self-limiting condition which responds well to laxatives. Chronic constipation occasionally ensues, particularly if there is a painful anal fissure. Acquired megacolon is produced by chronic constipation, and soiling results from liquid faeces percolating through these lumps in the rectum. It is not uncommon in childhood, with an incidence of 2 per cent in boys and just under 1 per cent in girls less than 7 years old. Most children acquire bowel control at around 2 years of age, so efforts at potty training before this age merely result in a conditioned reflex (i.e. defaecation when placed on the potty), which will cease when the child develops more bowel control. It is generally accepted that coercive bowel training during the first 18 months of life results in disappointments for the child and parents, which can easily become compounded by disapproval and hostility from parents.

Another manifestation of this type of inadequate potty training is encopresis (defined as normal defaecation in an inappropriate place), which is a distinct entity from constipation and soiling. Deep-seated emotional problems are common with encopresis, and sometimes remarkably rapid referral for advice will occur with very antisocial behaviour (e.g. using the fish tank or grand piano!). Help and advice will often be needed from social workers and child psychiatrists for this group of children who are difficult to manage.

Chronic constipation may have overlying emotional disturbances, but these tend to disappear once satisfactory treatment is instituted. It will be easier for the child to develop a normal relationship with his peers once his soiling has ceased.

Intussusception

Paul, aged 9 months, presented to his family doctor with a 16-hour history of screaming attacks during which he became pale. His parents commented that Paul was a fit child who had never had any similar episodes in the past and that they felt the screaming episodes were due to abdominal pain. Although he had vomited once, there had been no diarrhoea or constipation. The baby was slightly fractious and therefore difficult to examine. His abdomen was tender in all areas with a suggestion of a moderate sized periumbilical mass but a rectal examination was normal. He was sent to hospital for admission to the children's ward.

In view of these findings a nasogastric tube was passed and an intravenous infusion commenced. As Paul's condition was stable and there were no signs of peritonitis, a barium enema was performed (Fig. 5.17). This showed a hold-up of barium in the midtransverse colon with a filling defect, the typical appearances of intussusception.

An attempt was made to reduce the intussusception by hydrostatic pressure using barium solution which was run into the rectum from a bag 1 m above the table. The procedure was carried out under fluoroscopic control and produced a satisfactory reduction of the intussusception, confirmed by seeing a free flow of barium into the ileum.

Comment

Intussusception is the commonest cause of bowel obstruction in infancy, the usual site being the terminal ileum which invaginates and obstructs the caecum (Fig. 5.18). Children aged between 3 months and 2 years are most frequently affected, with the peak incidence occurring around 8 months of age. The cause of most intussusceptions is not known, although an association with viral infections and mesenteric adenitis has been suggested; on occasions an abnormality such as Meckel's diverticulum may be the predisposing factor.

The clinical features of intussusception are shown in Table 5.11. X-ray diagnosis is not necessary when the typical features are present.

Barium reduction is successful in 75 per cent of occasions when it is used. Open reduction

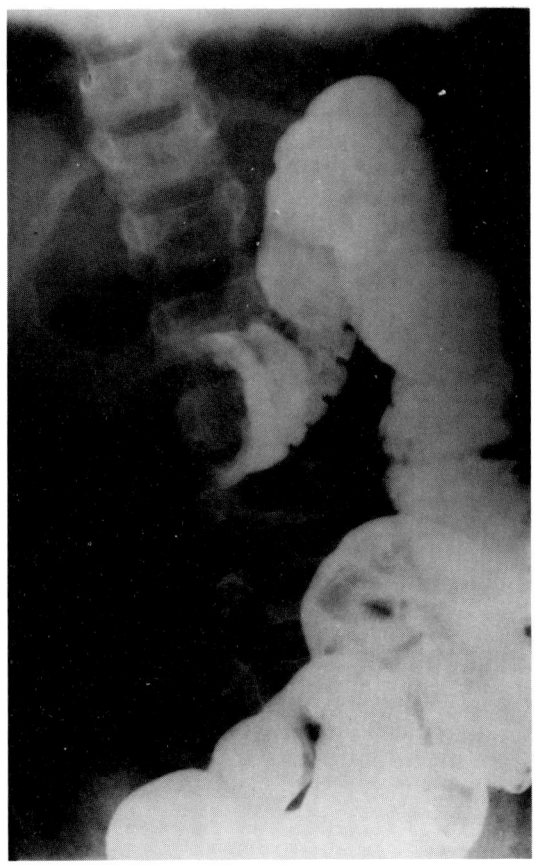

Fig. 5.17
Barium enema of intussusception

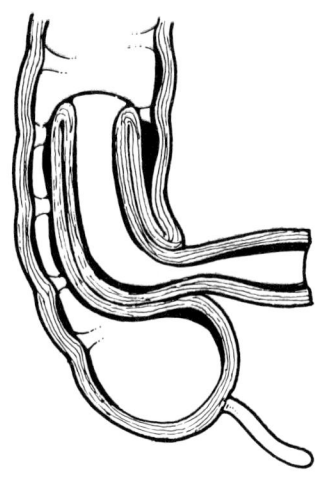

Fig. 5.18
Ileocolic intussusception

Table 5.11
Clinical features of an intussusception

History
Intermittent acute abdominal pain, with bouts of pallor, screaming and drawing up the legs
Vomiting (often absent initially)
Passage of blood and mucus in the stools
Bile-stained vomiting and constipation are late features of intestinal obstruction

Examination
Infant often febrile and unwell
Abdomen tender with a vague palpable mass
Blood and mucus on rectal examination

---

at laparotomy is indicated when this procedure fails to lead to resolution. Most surgeons feel that a history of more than 24 hours, an ill child and/or signs of peritonitis are indications for immediate surgery. An irreducible intussusception will need resection and end-to-end bowel anastomosis. Recurrences are sometimes seen following surgery or barium reduction, and the mortality is still appreciable due to late diagnosis and treatment.

Coeliac Disease

Celia, aged 9 months, presented with a four-month history of chronic diarrhoea, intermittent vomiting and failure to thrive. Her mother described her as 'an irritable child' who was seldom content even in the company of other children or adults. Several visits to the doctor had resulted in reassurance that there was no physical cause for Celia's disorder, which was likely to be behavioural in nature. Her mother had never been entirely convinced about this, as her 4-year-old daughter had always been a happy and contented child.

At examination a distended abdomen and gross muscle wasting were observed. Her tummy was large but her limbs were thin. A blood count showed a mild anaemia (Hb 9.8 g/dl) with a hypochromic blood film. In view of the failure to thrive, Celia was admitted to hospital for further sorting out. A jejunal biopsy was performed for suspected coeliac disease using a biopsy capsule (Figs. 5.19 and 5.20). The specimen obtained was examined under a dissecting microscope which revealed a lack of intestinal villi. Further examination of the fixed stained specimen showed a mucosa that was flat.

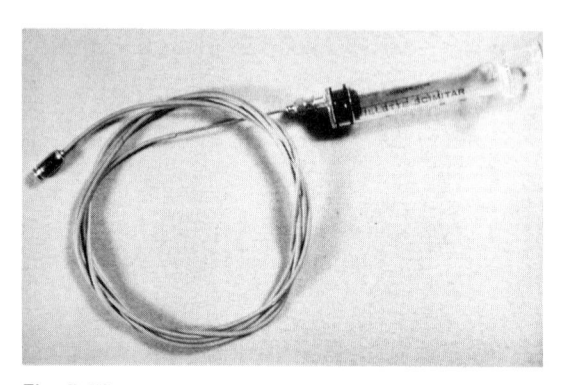

Fig. 5.19
Intestinal biopsy capsule

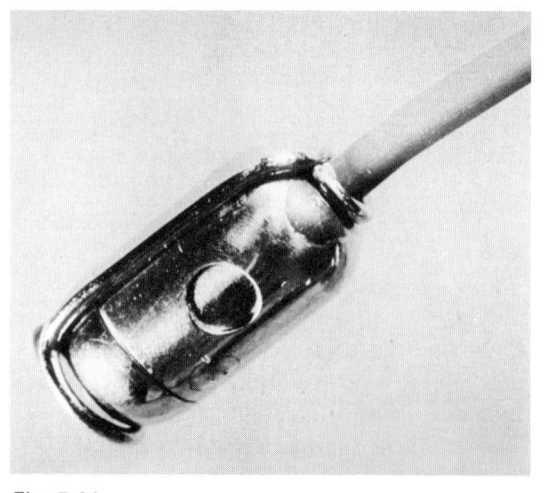

Fig. 5.20
Intestinal biopsy capsule head

Comment

Coeliac disease has an incidence of 1 in 2000 children, and was first described nearly 100 years ago. The small gut biopsy findings, first described in 1957, are typical of coeliac disease but, unfortunately, on rare occasions other conditions can cause similar findings (Table 5.12). It is thought that the alpha-gliadin fraction of gluten gives rise to an enteropathy by an immunological mechanism, and this leads to malabsorption because of loss of absorptive surface in the absence of villi.

Treatment is for life, so it is essential that the correct diagnosis be made. In view of the transient enteropathies listed, it is suggested by paediatric gastroenterologists that three jejunal biopsies are needed to finally confirm the diagnosis of coeliac disease, but in practice most paediatricians will undertake only two (initially and following a later gluten challenge).

The assistance of an experienced dietitian will always be needed for the exclusion of gluten from the diet (Fig. 5.21). Supervision is necessary in order to update dietary advice and to check compliance. The response to total removal of gluten is generally dramatic (Fig. 5.22). The prognosis is excellent, although there does seem to be a slightly increased risk of intestinal malignancy in adult life.

Table 5.12
Causes of a flat small bowel mucosa in children

Coeliac disease
Postgastroenteritis
Giardiasis
Cows' milk protein intolerance
Tropical sprue
Protein–calorie malnutrition
Acquired hypogammaglobulinaemia

Acute Appendicitis

Samantha, a lively 3 year old, refused to eat her breakfast and was unusually quiet and 'well behaved' for the first two hours of the day. Later that morning she vomited once and appeared to have some abdominal pain, so her mother telephoned the surgery. The

---

Obvious sources of gluten

    bread
    cakes
    pasta
    some breakfast cereals

Hidden gluten

    baby foods
    sausages
    fish fingers
    gravies and soups
    some tinned vegetables
    ice cream
    flavoured crisps

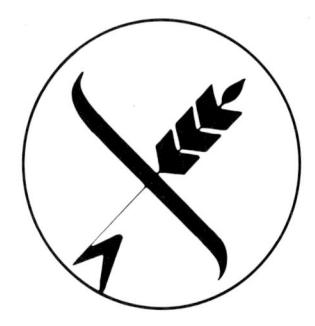

Symbol of Gluten-free Food

Fig. 5.21
Gluten-free diet (*From Milner AD & Hull D (1984)* Hospital Paediatrics. *Churchill Livingstone, Edinburgh, by courtesy of the publishers*)

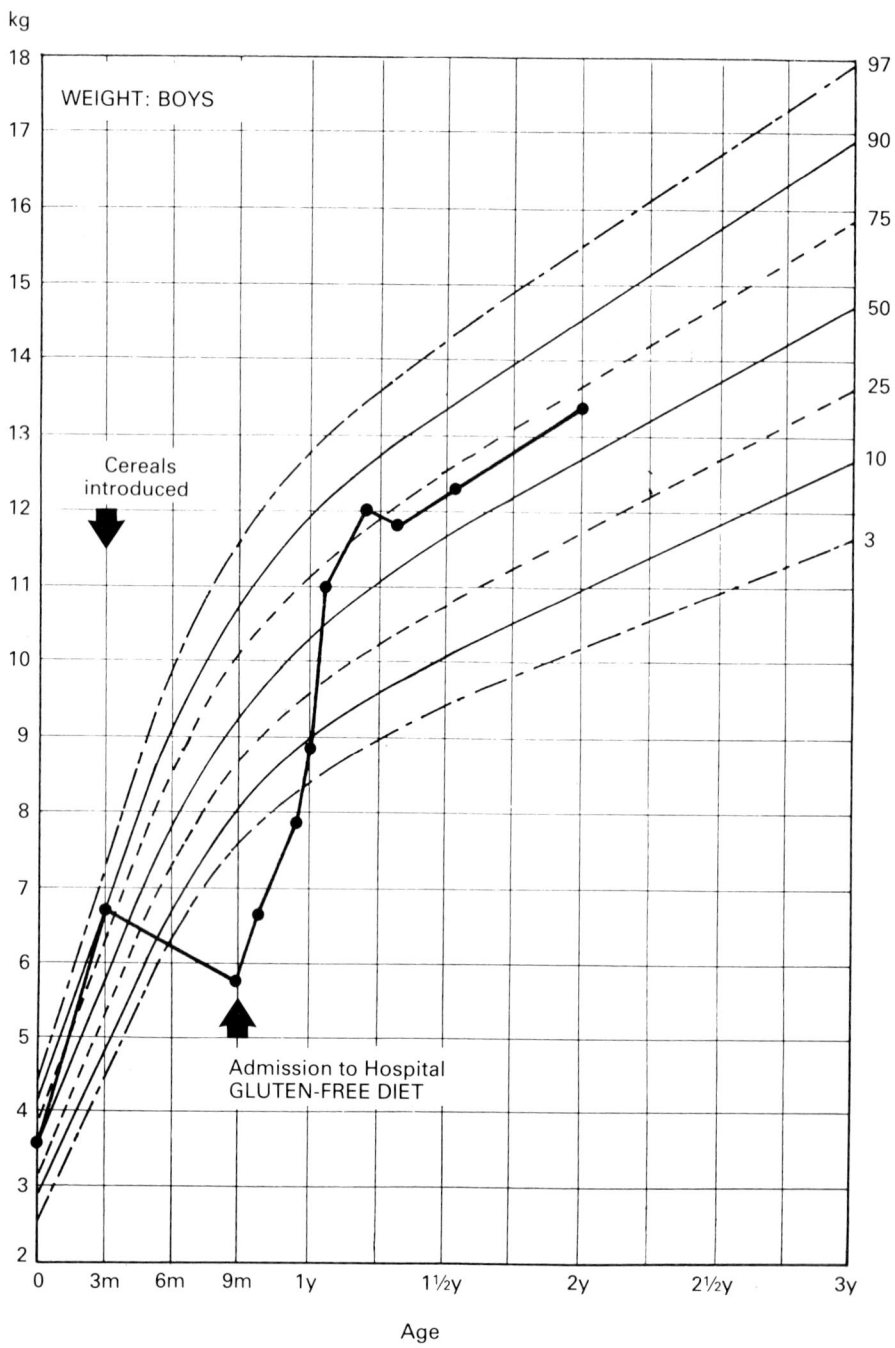

Fig. 5.22
Typical growth chart of child with coeliac disease

receptionist suggested phoning back later or bringing her up to the surgery the next day if things did not settle. By lunchtime Samantha was beginning to look decidedly seedy and unwell so her mother telephoned the surgery again and arranged a home visit by the doctor.

He found a pale, slightly febrile child with a tachycardia of 110 per minute. There were no features to suggest a respiratory infection or meningitis, but he noted slight abdominal distension associated with diffuse muscle guarding. The right side of the abdomen was tender on palpation.

Urgent transfer to hospital was arranged where the surgeons confirmed the physical signs and carried out a rectal examination which yielded no further information. At operation a grossly inflamed appendix, which had recently perforated, was found wrapped in a few loops of small bowel. An appendectomy was performed and intravenous antibiotics were commenced using gentamicin and metronidazole. Postoperative recovery was slow but uneventful, and the nasogastric tube was removed on the third day.

Comment

In the UK, 40 children a year still die from acute appendicitis, which can occur at any age after the first week of life. Teenagers are most commonly affected and diagnosis should not present difficulty at this age. Children under 3 years sometimes do not have any pain and the diagnosis can be very difficult. Gastroenteritis or a urinary infection are often diagnosed in error. In the older child, mesenteric adenitis and recurrent abdominal pain are the commonest alternatives. When atypical features are present, it is always worth thinking of other causes of acute abdominal pain (Table 5.13).

Complications can arise from appendicitis

Table 5.13

Acute abdominal pain in children

Common	Uncommon
Urinary tract infection	Diabetes mellitus
Gastroenteritis	Henoch–Schönlein
Lower lobe pneumonia	purpura
Constipation	Sickle cell crisis
Intussusception	
Mesenteric adenitis	

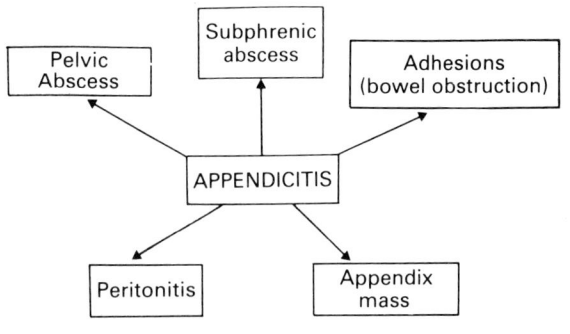

Fig. 5.23
Complications of appendicitis

(Fig. 5.23). Fortunately these are now less common with the advent of more effective postoperative antibiotics which are used if the appendix is gangrenous or if there is peritonitis. Metronidazole is particularly effective against anaerobic organisms implicated in intra-abdominal sepsis.

Early diagnosis and treatment favour a successful outcome to this potentially fatal disease. The overall mortality is less than 1 per cent.

Oesophageal Atresia

Ben was born at 35 weeks' gestation with a birth weight of 2.5 kg. His mother had had polyhydramnios during the last six weeks of the pregnancy and it was felt that this had precipitated premature delivery. The paediatrician at the birth found Ben to be in good shape with no evidence of asphyxia. Admission to the neonatal unit was arranged for observation.

Shortly after birth the nursing staff found Ben to be 'frothy' and in need of repeated sucking out. He appeared to produce a large volume of oral secretions. They had difficulty passing a nasogastric tube and, in view of the likely diagnosis of oesophageal atresia, an attempt was made to pass a large-bore orogastric tube (size 12G). This was unsuccessful because of an obstruction about 6 cm from the mouth at the T4 level (Fig. 5.24). Gas was present in the gut, so the diagnosis was oesophageal atresia with a tracheo-oesophageal fistula—the commonest variety. A double-lumen suction tube was sited in the pouch to aspirate secretions continuously. The next day he was taken to theatre for a thoracotomy to ligate the fistula in order to prevent acid gastric contents refluxing into the lungs (Fig. 5.25). In addition, a gastrostomy was

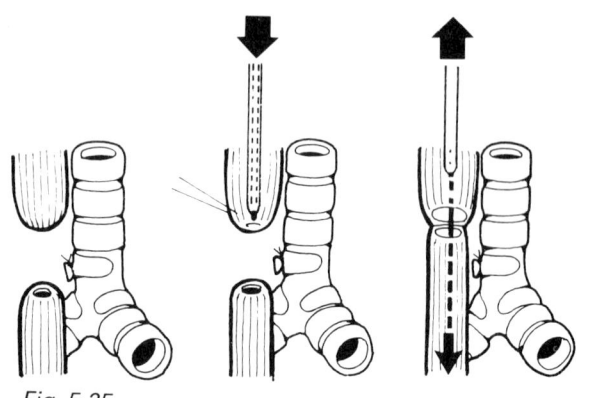

Fig. 5.25
Surgical correction of oesophageal atresia

made to enable feeding to commence. A second-stage repair was undertaken five weeks later, when the two ends of the oesophagus were joined together.

Comment

This serious congenital abnormality is relatively common, with an incidence of 1 in 2500. Maternal hydramnios can be associated with a number of fetal abnormalities, and it is always wise to pass a wide-bore tube at birth to diagnose cases of oesophageal atresia immediately, so that feeding is not commenced. Milk aspiration in the lungs can be serious!

About 87 per cent of cases have a tracheo-oesophageal fistula in addition to the oesophageal atresia, 8 per cent atresia alone with a wide gap between the ends, and 4 per cent

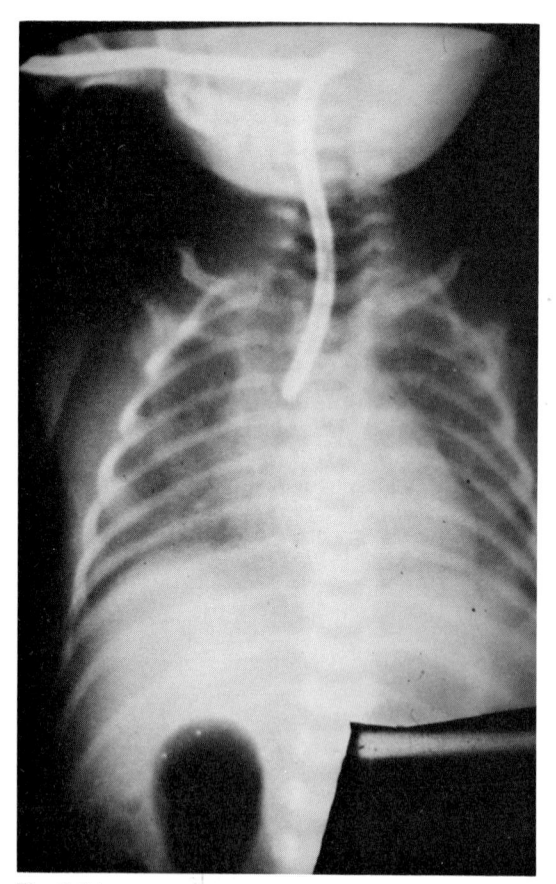

Fig. 5.24
X-ray of catheter in upper oesophageal pouch

the so-called H-type fistula with oesophageal atresia which presents at a later time with recurrent aspiration pneumonia. Other congenital abnormalities such as heart disease are frequently found in addition to oesophageal atresia.

Treatment involves ligation of the fistula and establishing oesophageal continuity, which is possible as a primary procedure in 75 per cent of cases. Where the gap is large, a second-stage procedure such as a colon transplant may be necessary at an older age.

Overall survival is influenced by time of diagnosis, associated anomalies, birth weight and skill of the surgical team. A 65 per cent overall survival is realistic.

6 Haematological diseases

Henoch–Schönlein purpura

Justin, a 7 year old, developed an upper respiratory infection which settled over several days. However, ten days later he developed joint pains in his knees and wrists as well as a florid rash over his arms, legs and buttocks. The eruption was purpuric in the form of large blotches with urticarial lesions on the legs (Fig. 6.1) and the buttocks (Fig. 6.2). As he had painful effusions of both knees, Justin found it very difficult to walk.

He was admitted to hospital for further assessment with a diagnosis of Henoch–Schönlein purpura (HSP). A throat swab failed to grow any pathogens, but regular ward testing of his urine revealed persistent haematuria. He remained reasonably well for 36 hours until he developed lower abdominal pain and a swollen painful left testis. The new houseman, who had just finished a surgical post, recognized an acute torsion of the testis and arranged for his surgical colleagues to see Justin. They arrived in the middle of a ward round, and after much discussion and deliberation it was felt that the testicle was not twisted, but was painful due to vasculitis as a result of the disease.

Fig. 6.1
Typical Henoch-Schönlein rash on legs

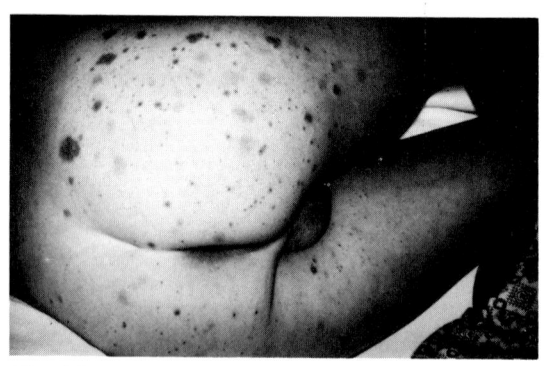

Fig. 6.2
Henoch-Schönlein rash on buttocks

Comment

HSP is a disease producing a diffuse vasculitis which can affect any part of the body. The disease process is probably triggered by a viral or bacterial infection and occurs in children aged from 2 to 10 years, being most frequent in preschool children.

Usually the florid rash, present on the extensor surfaces of the legs and buttocks, is diagnostic. Joint pain and local soft tissue swelling are frequent, as is abdominal pain due to bleeding into the bowel wall. Unfortunately, an intussusception can arise as a secondary phenomenon, so great care is needed in the management of abdominal pain. Blood in the stools can be seen in either situation. Testicular involvement is rare, but important to know about so that unnecessary surgery can be avoided. Analgesia alone is the usual treatment for HSP, but steroids may be useful in severe cases, particularly with marked abdominal pain.

The prognosis for the disease is good except in those children with permanent renal damage. Justin had evidence of nephritis, as do about a half of children with HSP. Proteinuria or haematuria will usually disappear, but follow-up is necessary in those when it persists as a few children will develop chronic renal failure. About 15 per cent of children entering a chronic dialysis or transplant programme have chronic renal failure secondary to HSP. Nevertheless the prognosis is good for the majority of children with this common illness.

Idiopathic Thrombocytopenic Purpura

Kate, a healthy 3 year old, had several major nosebleeds in three days which were difficult to control. She also developed a petechial rash on both legs with extensive bruising of her arms, legs and trunk. Her mother took her directly to the accident and emergency department because she felt sure her daughter had leukaemia.

Admission to the children's ward was arranged and investigations were undertaken. The bleeding time was prolonged and the blood count was entirely normal except for a very low platelet count of $6 \times 10^9/l$. Coagulation studies were within normal limits. A bone marrow examination was performed which showed increased numbers of megakaryoctes and normal numbers of red and white cell precursors. Kate's parents were reassured that she did not have leukaemia.

Kate was treated with a course of oral prednisolone, and although her platelet count remained static for several weeks her bruises faded. By eight weeks her platelet count was slowly beginning to increase and no new bruises or petechiae were appearing. She was discharged home after a week and was followed as an outpatient. By three months her platelet count had returned to normal.

Comment

Kate had idiopathic thrombocytopenic purpura (ITP), one of the commoner haematological disorders of children which is frequently precipitated by viral infections such as rubella. The thrombocytopenia is due to excessive platelet destruction by the reticuloendothelial system, especially the spleen, which leads to increased platelet production by the bone marrow. It appears that antiplatelet IgG antibodies attach themselves to platelets, which render them susceptible to destruction by the spleen.

ITP is the commonest cause of thrombocytopenia in children, but the diagnosis must be made by exclusion of other disease. A careful drug history is important before other tests are carried out since some drugs, particularly sulphonamides, cause thrombocytopenia. Most paediatricians would recommend a bone marrow examination to exclude an infiltration or an aplasia of the marrow producing thrombocytopenia, although anaemia and neutropenia would usually be present in these conditions.

About 90 per cent of children have acute ITP, which is a self-limiting condition, usually disappearing within three months. Although steroids have little effect on the platelet count, many paediatricians use them if the platelet count is very low to prevent life-threatening bleeding. Emergency splenectomy is occasionally undertaken for a serious cerebral haemorrhage. Some cases of chronic ITP respond to splenectomy but there is always the risk of later bacterial septicaemia. Fortunately, only 1 per cent of all cases have major haemorrhage, so the prognosis is excellent for most children.

Haemophilia

Carl, a 10-year-old boy with moderately severe haemophilia, knocked his right knee on the handlebar of his bicycle whilst chasing his brother. He was just able to limp home to his mother, who found his knee to be very swollen. She administered 400 units of factor VIII concentrate (which she stored in her 'fridge) intravenously via a butterfly needle.

In view of the swelling she took Carl to the regional haemophilia centre which was 20 miles away. It was decided to admit Carl for further treatment and an orthopaedic surgeon was asked to review him. He aspirated the knee under local anaesthetic with a wide-bore needle before any more treatment was given. Factor VIII concentrate (half-life eight hours) was given three times a day to maintain Carl's plasma levels at above 25 per cent of normal for the next few days. A physiotherapist initially taught Carl passive quadriceps exercises, and then helped him with mobilization on crutches. He was able to go home after a week.

Comment

Haemophilia, a congenital deficiency of factor VIII, is present in 1 in 10 000 male infants and is inherited as a sex-linked recessive disorder. Christmas disease, due to factor IX deficiency, is a much less common disorder. Manifestations of haemophilia become apparent around 6 months of age when the infant is becoming mobile, unless presentation has followed circumcision at birth.

Initial clotting studies will reveal a prolonged partial thromboplastin time, so specific measurements of factors VIII and IX will be needed (Table 6.1). Screening should be

Table 6.1

Screening tests for disorders of coagulation

Whole blood clotting time:
prolonged in severe disorders, but little used
Prothrombin time (PT):
a test of tissue thromboplastin production which involves liver coagulation proteins but not factors VIII or IX
Partial thromboplastin time (PTT):
a test of blood thromboplastin production which involves factors VIII and IX

Direct assay of the specific factors is performed to make the definitive diagnosis of haemophilia or Christmas disease

carried out in male infants with bruising thought to be due to non-accidental injury as well as in children with soft tissue or joint bleeding, as unusual presentations are possible. Factor VIII levels correlate well with clinical manifestations (Table 6.2). Joint haemorrhages are the commonest feature of the severe disease and may lead to joint damage (Fig. 6.3). Bleeding into soft tissues or muscle is common too, but renal or gastrointestinal bleeding is less often seen.

Table 6.2

Severity of haemophilia realted to factor VIII levels

Factor VIII level (% normal)	Features
25–50%	Asymptomatic or bleeding after major trauma
5–25%	Mild haemophilia with prolonged bleeding after injury or surgery
1–5%	Moderate haemophilia with frequent bleeding after trivial trauma
<1%	Severe haemophilia with spontaneous bleeding and involvement of joints and muscles

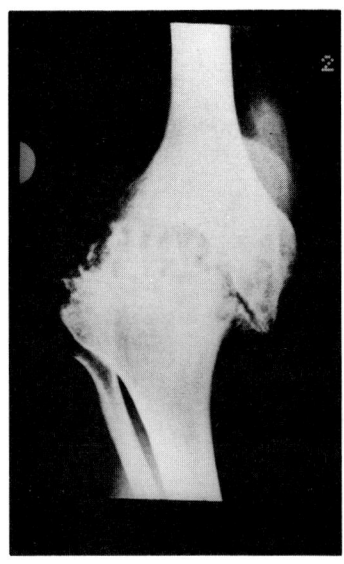

Fig. 6.3
Destruction of knee joint

Management involves a multidisciplinary approach to the child (Fig. 6.4), with emphasis on home treatment by parents for minor bleeds. Factor VIII concentrates are replacing cryoprecipitate, as storage and administration

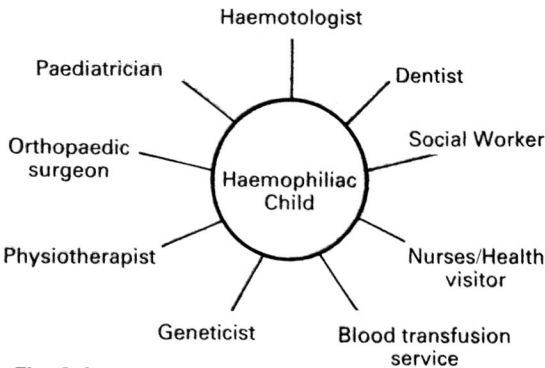

Fig. 6.4
Multidisciplinary team for haemophiliac child

are easier. The dose depends on the nature of the injury, but is easily calculated because 1 ml of normal plasma has 1 unit of activity. Antibody inhibition of factor VIII will present treatment problems for a minority of children but fortunately hepatitis is uncommon. Anxieties about the risks of acquired immune deficiency syndrome (AIDS) may need to be quelled.

Screening of families enables 85 per cent of carriers to be detected and antenatal diagnosis of haemophilia is now possible from umbilical vein blood samples taken after sexing of the unborn infant by fetoscopy. Haemophilia breeds true, so families with more severely affected individuals who are handicapped may be more keen on intervention during a pregnancy. Full information must be provided to enable families to make informed decisions themselves. The prognosis is improving as treatment becomes more satisfactory and supplies of factor VIII increase.

Iron Deficiency Anaemia

Fay, an 18-month-old child, was periodically seen at home by her health visitor who thought she looked pale. Birth weight had been 2.40 kg at term, and she had been bottle fed until 4 months of age when weaning was commenced. There was no history of anaemia in the other four children, the eldest of whom refused to attend school. Various concerns about the care of the children had been raised over the previous few months and the social worker and health visitor kept a careful watch on the home. Both had suspicions about the father swapping milk tokens for cigarettes at the local newsagent.

Fay was taken to see her family doctor who found signs of pallor without any history to suggest any underlying illness. A blood count revealed a haemoglobin of 8.8 g/dl (normal range 10.7–13.1 g/dl) with a hypochromic microcytic picture but with normal platelets and white cells. A course of oral iron in the form of ferrous sulphate mixture was given and the blood count repeated after three weeks. The haemoglobin levels had only risen to 9.5 g/dl with a 2 per cent reticulocyte response but in fact very little ferrous sulphate had been used as the first bottle prescribed was nearly full! The health visitor initially undertook daily home visits to ensure adequate drug compliance and a three-month course of treatment was given. The blood count taken two weeks later showed a satisfactory response to treatment. The haemoglobin rose steadily and a month later was 12.0 g/dl.

Comment

Iron deficiency anaemia is by far the commonest cause of anaemia in children, having a

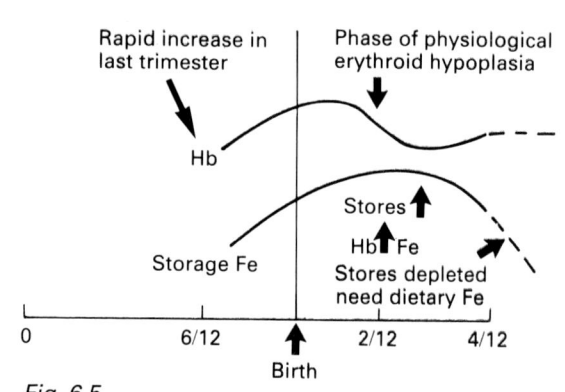

Fig. 6.5
Pathogenesis of iron deficiency in infancy

maximum incidence at between 6 months and 3 years. Surveys have shown that as many as two-thirds of lastborn children from deprived inner city areas will be affected.

Most iron stores in the neonate are held in the form of circulating haemoglobin, so low birth weight or neonatal anaemia will predispose to iron deficiency because iron stores become prematurely exhausted (Fig. 6.5). Milk, the natural food of infants, contains very little iron unless it is fortified, and iron intake will be low until weaning on to solids is complete. The factors predisposing the infant to iron deficiency are summarized in Table 6.3.

Diagnosis is made from the history, examination and blood count. Routine measurements of serum iron, ferritin or lead levels etc. should be avoided as they are unhelpful and cause chronic bleeding of health service resources! The history should alert one to the possibility of blood loss. Atypical features or failure to respond to treatment will indicate

Table 6.3
Causes of iron deficiency in infants

Poor intake	Low stores	Blood loss
Dietary lack	Late weaning	Meckel's diverticulum
Anorexia	Low birth weight	Reflux oesophagitis
Coeliac disease (malabsorption of iron)	Multiple pregnancy	Repeated venepuncture

the small number of children who need further investigations. Non-compliance is the commonest cause of treatment failure, but there are other causes of a hypochromic anaemia besides iron deficiency (Table 6.4).

Table 6.4
Causes of a hypochromic anaemia other than iron deficiency

Thalassaemia
Chronic infection
Lead poisoning
Sideroblastic anaemia

Three months' treatment with oral iron provides enough to correct the anaemia and replenish iron stores. After a lag period of a week the haemoglobin level should increase by 1 g/dl every ten days. Since most children have anaemia secondary to dietary deficiency, the prognosis is excellent.

Leukaemia

Kathryn, an 8 year old, had been unwell for six weeks with weight loss, tiredness and marked bruising over her arms and chest. A blood count taken by her GP showed the following results:

>   Hb 6.2 g/dl
>   WBC $10 \times 10^9/l$ with 50 per cent blast cells
>   Platelets $20 \times 10^9/l$

The peripheral blood film revealed the presence of blast cells (Fig. 6.6). Physical examination showed splenomegaly, pallor and a few retinal haemorrhages. She was referred to the paediatric outpatient clinic with a provisional diagnosis of leukaemia, where the physical findings were confirmed. Some bony tenderness was present in the left hand, and a skeletal survey showed bony destruction of

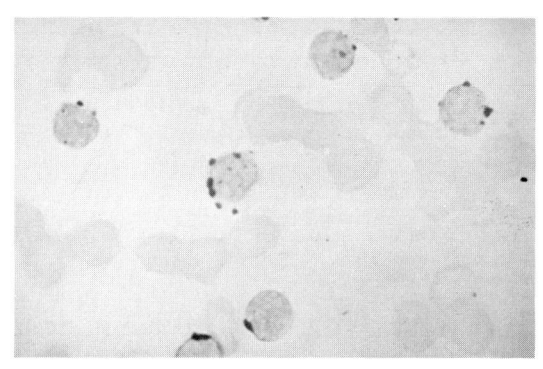

Fig. 6.6
Blood film in acute lymphatic leukaemia

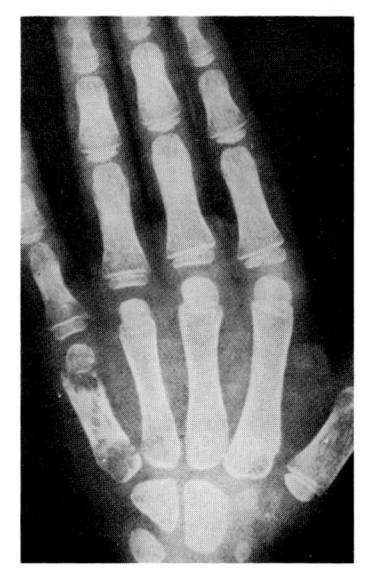

Fig. 6.7
Bony destruction of fifth metacarpal

the fifth metacarpal (Fig. 6.7) and transverse bands of increased and decreased density in the metaphyses of the femur.

A bone marrow examination revealed numerous blast cells typical of acute lymphoblastic leukaemia (ALL), the commonest variety of leukaemia in children (85 per cent), and she was admitted to hospital for treatment.

Comment

The disease is caused by proliferation of a clone of lymphoid stem cells—and up to 1 kg (10^{12} cells) may be present. 'Surface markers' can be detected on these blast cells using immunological techniques and help in assessing the prognosis. Markers typical of T cells (19 per cent) or B cells (1 per cent) indicate that there will be a poor response to treatment. The remainder of cases (80 per cent) fall into the common ALL group with a better prognosis. The disease presents with bruising (from thrombocytopenia), infections (from neutropenia) and tiredness (from anaemia), and with bone pain.

There are about 350 new cases of leukaemia each year in children under 15 years in the UK. Results of treatment are best where a regional oncology centre is involved, and Kathryn's care was shared between the district hospital and the regional centre. Treatment is complex and involves drugs and radiotherapy. Unfortunately, after a few weeks' treatment Kathryn's sister came out in the rash of chickenpox. This is a serious infection in immunosuppressed children. Depression of bone marrow and immune system by a combination of drugs and disease render Kathryn likely to have an overwhelming chickenpox/zoster infection without prophylaxis with hyperimmune zoster immunoglobulin.

Other complications of the disease sometimes arise, but about one-third to one-half of children will be cured. The aims of treatment must be to maintain the child in permanent remission, and returned to full health once the maintenance schedule has been completed. Side effects of the treatment are numerous (Table 6.5). As with any chronic disease in children, the importance of a good relationship between family and medical, nursing and social work staff is crucial to the success of these plans. The improvement in prognosis during the last decade is best shown by calculating the percentage of children alive in first remission, as even one relapse means there is no chance of permanent cure.

Sickle Cell Disease

Leonora, a 4 year old with sickle cell disease, was admitted to hospital with a 12-hour history of severe back pains and vomiting. Her lower lumbar spine was diffusely tender and she had a low grade fever. Several similar episodes had occurred during the preceding 12 months. In spite of her moderate anaemia and small size, Leonora was generally a well child who attended her local day nursery without too many days missed through illness. The only manifestations of disease were a slightly

Table 6.5

Side effects of treatment of acute lymphoblastic leukaemia

Drugs	Anorexia, vomiting, constipation, neuropathy, alopecia, oral ulceration, renal and hepatic damage
Radiotherapy	Alopecia, vomiting, lethargy and drowsiness Mild intellectual impairment, pituitary damage
Immunosuppression	An increase in bacterial infection (especially Gram-negative organisms) Severe infections caused by herpes simplex, varicella, cytomegalovirus, measles, pneumocystis and candida

enlarged spleen and an abnormal skull x-ray, which showed a 'hair on end' appearance of the frontal bone.

She was admitted to hospital and needed intravenous fluids to correct dehydration, morphine for pain relief and oxygen. Her pain settled over the next few days and it was felt she had had an infarctive crisis, the most common reason for hospital admission in such children. After discharge, Leonora continued outpatient follow-up, taking prophylactic folate supplements and penicillin.

Comment

The WHO estimates that 80 000 children a year die from sickle cell disease (SCD), which is a disease found in Negros of Central African stock, who have a carrier rate for the sickle gene of around 20 per cent. Autosomal dominant inheritance is the mechanism of transmission, and SCD occurs when both parents carry the sickle cell trait (Fig. 6.8). The sickle gene leads to production of an abnormal haemoglobin (HbS) due to a single amino-acid substitution in the beta globulin chain, and this can be easily identified *in vitro* by haemoglobin electrophoresis. Heterozygotes (sickle cell trait) have 40 per cent of their haemoglobin in the form of HbS, so they are asymptomatic unless involved in deep sea diving or mountaineering, when their PaO_2 may drop to very low levels and induce sickling. In homozygotes (SCD) the rigid deformed red cells have a shortened survival, resulting in anaemia and obstruction of small vessels with infarction.

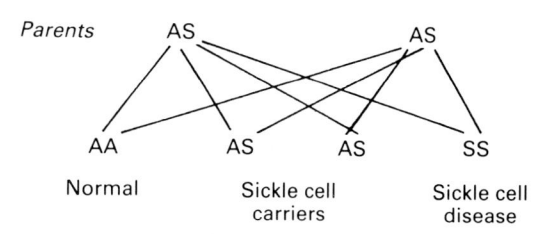

Fig. 6.8
Inheritance of sickle cell disease

Laboratory diagnosis of sickle trait and SCD is easy (Table 6.6), but the advantages of neonatal screening have yet to be proven. Genetic advice should be available to all sickle trait individuals, as SCD treatment is still far from satisfactory. SCD can now be identified antenatally in early pregnancy by analysis of DNA from amniotic cells or trophoblast.

Management of SCD includes supportive measures with recognition and treatment of infection and specific prophylaxis against pneumococcal septicaemia by polyvalent vaccine or penicillin. Children with SCD infarct their spleens and are particularly susceptible to severe bacterial infections. Folic acid deficiency which may arise from the high red cell turnover should be prevented by regular supplementation. Specific management of infarc-

Table 6.6
Laboratory diagnosis of sickle cell anaemia (trait and disease)

	Trait	**Disease**
Haemoglobin	Normal	Low
Blood film	Normal	Sickle cells present
Sickling test	Positive	Positive
Hb electrophoresis	HbS and HbA present	HbS without HbA

tive crises is not available, but hyperbaric oxygen can be beneficial in life-threatening situations. The pregnant patient with SCD will need top-up or partial exchange blood transfusions.

Many children still die during the first ten years of life from renal failure, cerebral infarction or overwhelming sepsis, but the prognosis is improving and so some adults now reach their fourth and fifth decades.

7 Endocrine diseases

Short Stature

Stephanie was seen at a growth clinic at 13 years of age with short stature. Her height was about 2.5 standard deviations below the mean for age, as was her weight. It was noted that her parents' heights were on the 10th and 50th centiles and the routine examination was normal. A few initial investigations were carried out to exclude a thyroid or renal disorder and the chromosome karyotype was checked. These results were all normal but Stephanie's bone age was delayed at only 8 years. Long-term follow-up over a number of years revealed the typical picture of growth delay with her final height achieved at 21 years (Fig. 7.1).

The short stature combined with the absence of secondary sexual characteristics led to teasing at school and psychological problems, and these resolved at around 18 years, the age of menarche. The height difference between Stephanie and her peers was accentuated by the adolescent growth spurt, which her classmates had at between 11 and 14 years while Stephanie was still at a low prepubertal annual growth rate of 3 cm per year (Fig. 7.2). Nevertheless Stephanie continued growing for several years after her friends had stopped, achieving a final height of 1.55 m, without specific treatment.

Comment

Children with short stature are brought to medical attention by parents more readily than excessively tall individuals. Generally, short stature is less socially acceptable in boys than girls, especially in teenagers who are likely to have associated delayed puberty. Since 1 in 30 children have a height below the 3rd centile, and most are normal, the plotting of an individual height and weight at a single time will be of limited value. Repeat measurements six months later will give a growth velocity, and, in children with a low growth velocity, further evaluation will be necessary (Table 7.1). This includes the accurate assessment of pubertal status in older chil-

Table 7.1
Evaluation of a short child

Enquiry	Parental heights
	Birth weight
	Home circumstances
Assessment	Current height and weight
	Body proportions
	Sexual development
	Associated anomalies
	Growth velocity
Investigation	Bone age (for skeletal maturity)
	Skull x-ray (for a pituitary lesion)
	Chromosome studies (for Turner's syndrome in girls)
	Thyroid function (for hypothyroidism)
	Growth hormone release (for pituitary deficiency) especially if growth velocity low

84 CLINICAL CASES IN PAEDIATRICS

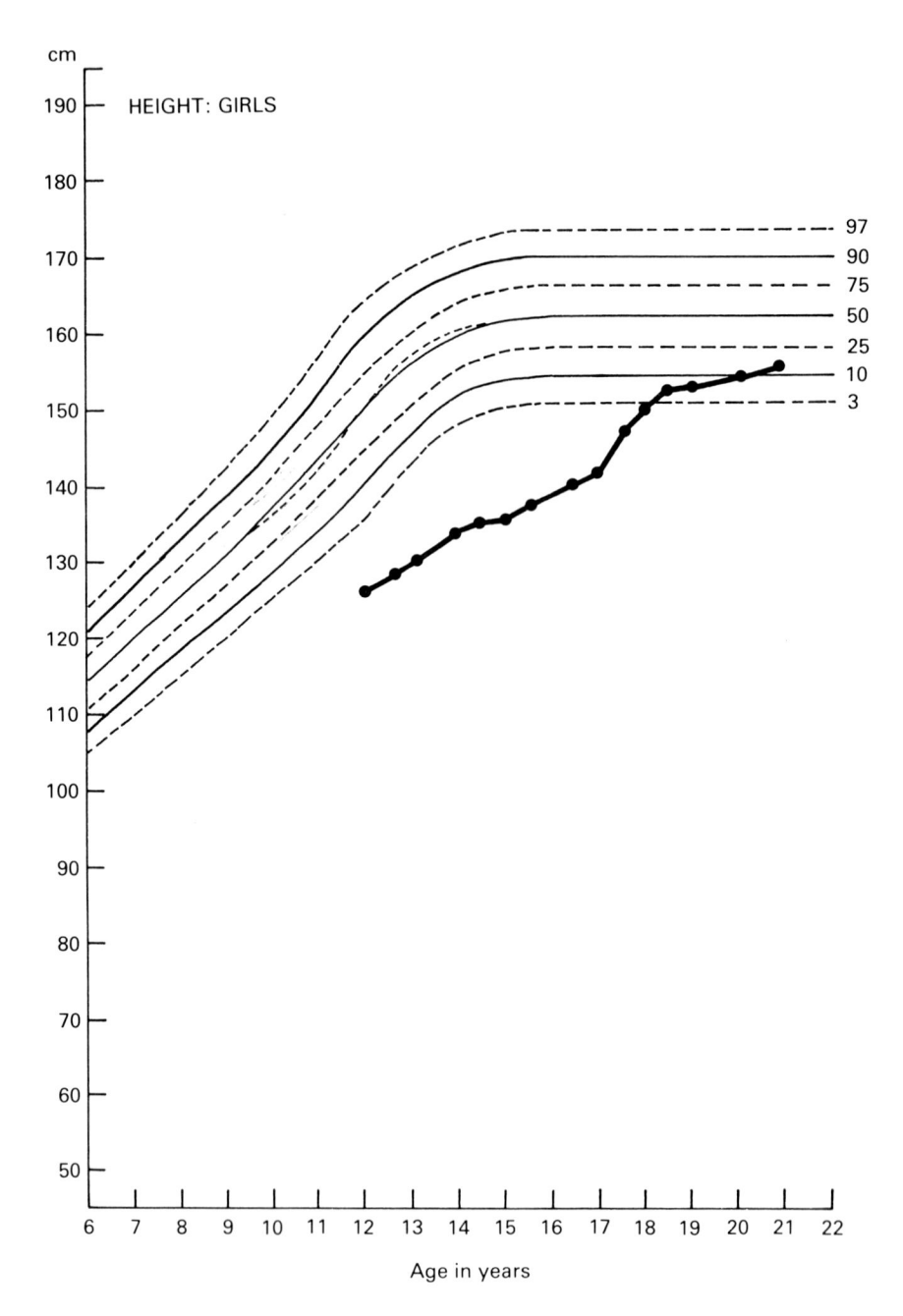

Fig. 7.1
Growth chart in growth delay

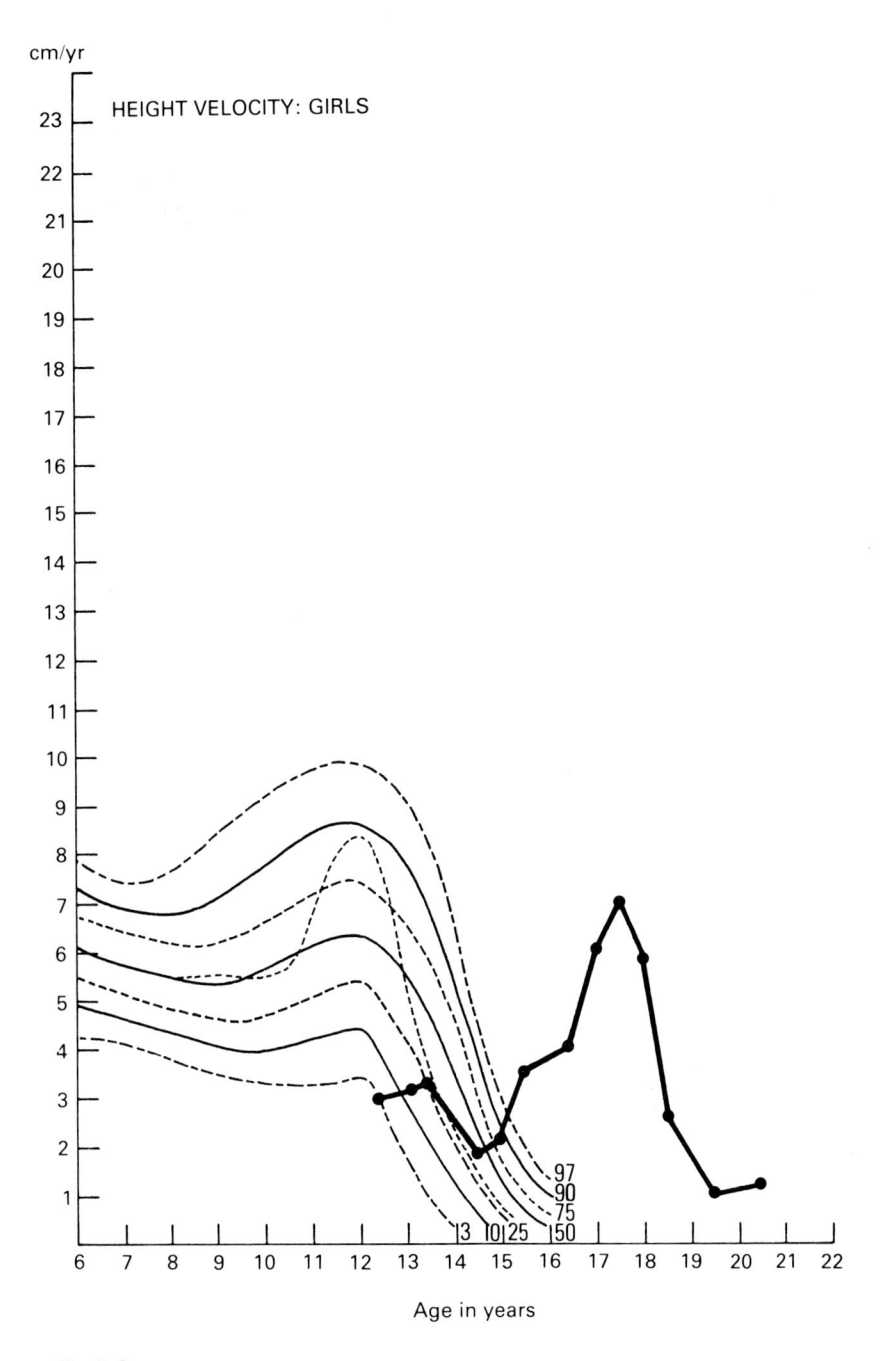

Fig. 7.2
Growth velocity in growth delay

dren. Full details of these are on the widely used Tanner growth charts.

There is a wide range of disorders causing short stature, but more than 80 per cent are variants of normal growth patterns (Table 7.2). If both parents are small their offspring will be of similar size, as mid-parental height has a correlation of 0.75 with final height of a child (genetic short stature). Growth delay is a diagnosis made by exclusion of pathological conditions and by careful follow-up. The unfortunate child with a combination of both genetic short stature and growth delay will be very short and no specific treatment will be of help. Short stature due to pathological disorders is most likely due to psychosocial causes, Turner's syndrome or a systemic disorder such as coeliac disease. Acceleration of growth in an improved social environment is diagnostic of the emotionally deprived child.

Psychological support is needed for all children and families with short stature. Early diagnosis and treatment are important for the less common diseases causing short stature (e.g. coeliac disease or growth hormone deficiency) if full growth potential is to be achieved.

Table 7.2
Variations in the normal pattern of growth

Genetic short stature
Height is normal when allowance is made for the parents' height
Growth delay (slow tempo of growth)
Height normal for bone age rather than chronological age
Puberty is delayed, growth continues for longer and eventual height is normal
A combination of the above
Such children are very small, particularly in relation to their pubertal peers

Diabetes Mellitus

Janet, a 10-year-old child with diabetes of 7 years' duration, was referred to the children's diabetic clinic for long-term management, as the family had just moved into the area. She was giving herself a once-daily insulin injection before breakfast, using a mixture of two highly purified porcine insulins (Actrapid and Monotard), but she was waking at night with thirst and nocturia. Her parents had not had much success in improving her symptoms by adjusting her insulin dosage and they were adamant that her injection routine should not be altered. Blood glucose control was assessed indirectly by urine testing for sugar semiquantitatively with Clinitest tablets but nearly all the tests were negative.

It was decided to introduce home blood glucose monitoring, and capillary blood samples were obtained from finger pricks (Fig. 7.3) to

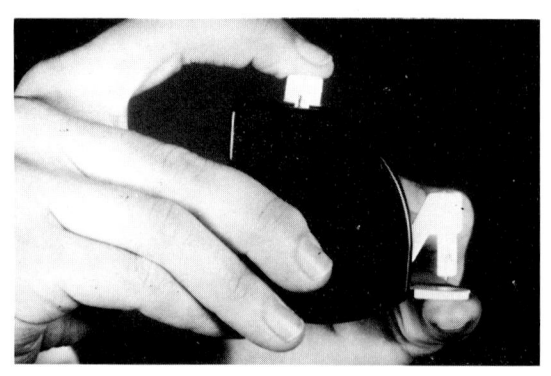

Fig. 7.3
Automatic device for finger pricking (*Autolet-Owen-Mumford Ltd*)

measure blood glucose levels with BM-Test Glycemie 20–800 sticks (Fig. 7.4). During the introduction of this new technique a diabetic health visitor was able to give regular tuition at home. The parents were surprised to find late night and fasting glucose values were often above 20 mmol/l and they began to

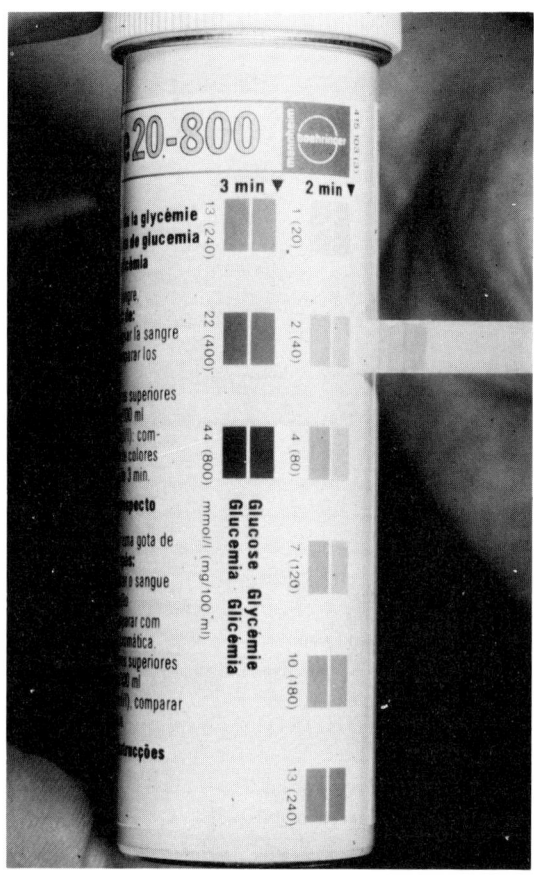

Fig. 7.4
BM-Test Glycemie 20-800 sticks (*Boehringer-Mannheim Ltd*)

realize that a second injection of insulin would be beneficial. At the next outpatient visit Janet was switched to a twice-daily insulin regimen which improved her diabetic control. The parents were surprised that their daughter preferred twice-daily insulin, but she felt better in herself on this regimen.

Comment

Diabetes is common (Table 7.3). The prevalence in the UK is 1 in 700 children up to 16

Table 7.3
Prevalence of diabetes in Great Britain

	No. of patients
On diet/tablets	270 000
On insulin	70 000
Total	340 000

I.e. 1 patient on insulin to every 4 on diet/tablets.

years of age and 1 in 300 under 26 years, and there are strong indications that the incidence is rising. Insulin treatment, which is necessary for all diabetic children, has now been available for more than 60 years; before this, the life expectancy for children averaged only 30 months after diagnosis. Microvascular complications secondary to prolonged hyperglycaemia include retinopathy, neuropathy and nephropathy. They are seen 10–20 years after diagnosis, and produce a tenfold increase in the mortality rate of young diabetics and a reduction in life expectancy to three-quarters of normal. Optimal blood glucose control should help to reduce the chances of these devastating side effects such as blindness or chronic renal failure.

Janet's unhelpful urine test results may have been due to a high renal threshold for glucose, poor testing technique or falsification of results. Many teenage children prefer regular home blood glucose monitoring to urine testing. Another aspect of management which needed checking was injection technique, with emphasis on the use of suitable sites (Fig. 7.5). When the child repeatedly uses the same place for each injection, fat hypertrophy of subcutaneous tissue will result (Fig. 7.6) and lead to erratic insulin absorption. Lipoatrophy at injection sites is an immunologically mediated phenomenon which is seen during the administration of impure bovine insulins that are rarely used for treating diabetic

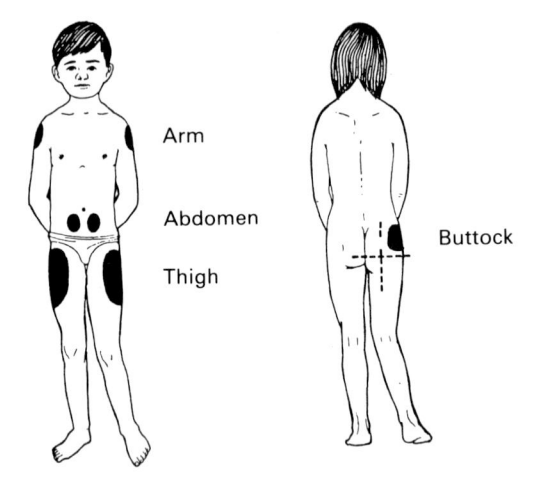

Fig. 7.5
Injection sites in diabetic child

children in developed countries. The problem does not occur with the highly purified porcine or human insulins which are the treatment of choice for diabetic children.

Hypoglycaemia is feared by children and their parents (Fig. 7.7). The frequency of this complication of treatment should be minimized by careful education of families and by ensuring sensible insulin regimens which avoid excessive insulin dosages. The future lies in the development of more flexible systems for delivering insulin and the prevention of the disease once the aetiology has been fully unravelled.

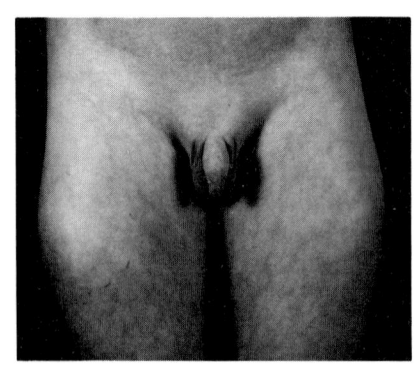

Fig. 7.6
Lipohypertrophy of thighs

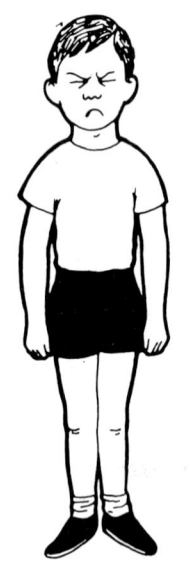

Fig. 7.7
Hypoglycaemia

Hypothyroidism

Ranjit was a 3-week-old baby, born following a normal pregnancy, labour and delivery with a birth weight of 3.40 kg. The health visitor had been contacted by the hospital when he was 2 weeks old because the neonatal thyroid screening test performed on the Guthrie blood sample was abnormal. The baby appeared well but the parents felt he was a little slow to feed. After a long explanation to the parents (who spoke English), an outpatient appointment was arranged for the next day.

The paediatrician learnt that the parents, who were unrelated, originally came from Sri Lanka and that there was no family history of thyroid disorder or goitrogen ingestion during the pregnancy. There were no abnormal findings when the baby was examined. Investigations showed that the bone age of the knee was delayed; serum thyroxine was 58 nmol/l (normal > 100 nmol/l); and TSH 455 mU/l (normal < 10 mU/l). As with all laboratory

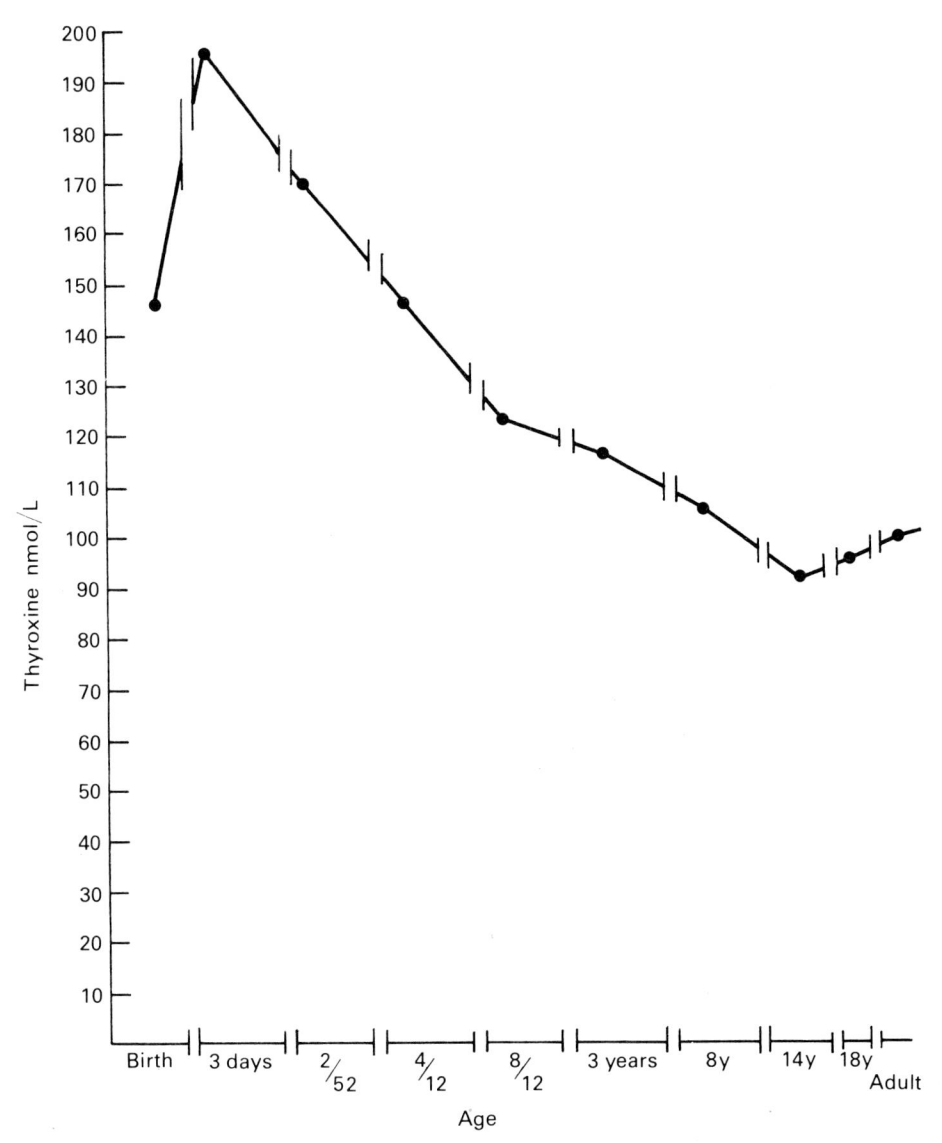

Fig. 7.8
Mean thyroxine levels in children

tests in children the reference values appropriate for age are needed to interpret the results (Fig. 7.8). These results confirmed primary hypothyroidism.

Once-daily L-thyroxine (6 µg/kg body weight per day) was commenced and regular follow-up arranged. At 1 year of age, tri-iodothyronine (which has a short half-life) was temporarily substituted for thyroxine. All treatment was stopped for a few days and thyroid function checked to exclude transient hypothyroidism and confirm the need for life-long treatment. This again showed a low serum thyroxine and a high TSH, indicating permanent primary hypothyroidism.

Comment

Screening programmes for congenital hypothyroidism were initially developed in 1974, and have since revealed an incidence of 1 in 3500 live births in the UK. Typical features of hypothyroidism (Fig. 7.9) are present in fewer than 10 per cent of newborns detected by screening procedures. Before screening was available, diagnosis was made at a later age following presentation with short stature; the typical facies, as shown in a 3-month child (Fig. 7.10); or developmental delay in early childhood. Unfortunately, such children with delayed diagnosis are likely to suffer permanent brain damage, remaining mentally retarded in spite of treatment. About 25 per cent of such children will have an IQ less than 70 and will need special education.

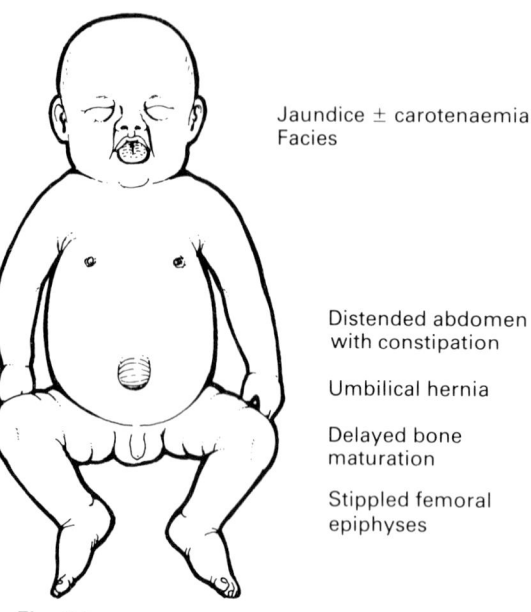

In the fetus the pituitary–thyroid axis is functioning by 20 weeks' gestation. Hypothyroidism is nearly always secondary to a defect in the thyroid gland itself, an ectopic gland being the most common abnormality. The loss of feedback of T_3 and T_4 on the anterior pituitary results in excess TSH production. Unfortunately, maternal thyroxine cannot cross the placenta, so the fetus is not protected *in utero*. Early treatment during the first month, however, appears to prevent most later handicap.

Fig. 7.9
Features of hypothyroidism

- Jaundice ± carotenaemia
- Facies
- Distended abdomen with constipation
- Umbilical hernia
- Delayed bone maturation
- Stippled femoral epiphyses

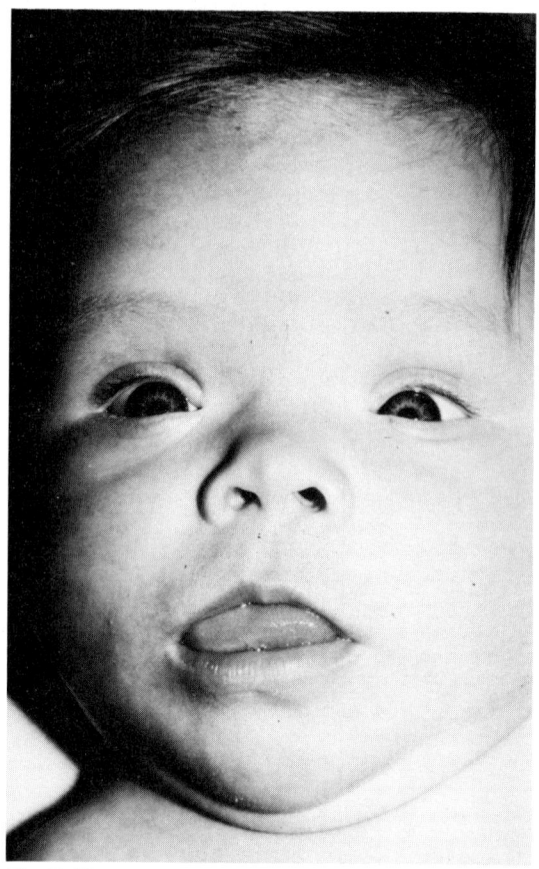

Fig. 7.10
Facies of hypothyroid child

The general principles of biochemical screening, which are as applicable to amino acid disorders as hypothyroidism are shown in Table 7.4. It is hoped that late presentation of congenital hypothyroidism will no longer occur.

Table 7.4

Principles of screening for a disease

The natural history of the untreated disease should be well known
The untreated disease should be a significant one
It should be treatable
Facilities for diagnosis and treatment should be available
The screening test should have a high sensitivity and specificity
The whole exercise should be economically justifiable

Congenital Adrenal Hyperplasia

Daniel, aged 3 weeks, was admitted to hospital at 3:00 a.m. with a feeding problem. He had been slow to feed and had had several episodes of vomiting during the previous 48 hours. Routine observations were carried out during the night, but when he was reassessed the next morning by another doctor he was found moribund and dehydrated with no localized signs of infection. He was treated with intravenous plasma and antibiotics after an infection screen had been carried out.

The electrolyte results revealed profound hyponatraemia with a moderate hyperkalaemia (Table 7.5) so his infusion was changed to physiological (normal) saline. Further blood was taken for an urgent 17-OH-progesterone level, and a bolus of hydrocortisone given. Later that day an ultrasound scan of the kidneys and renal tract excluded any hydronephrosis or bladder outlet obstruction. In the early evening the 17-OH-progesterone level result was found to be 488 nmol/l (normal < 15 nmol/l), confirming the diagnosis of salt-losing congenital adrenal hyperplasia.

Table 7.5

Daniel's electrolyte results (normal ranges in parentheses)

Urea	16 mmol/l (normal 3.3–7.5)
Sodium	104 mmol/l (135–143)
Potassium	6.3 mmol/l (3.3–4.7)
Bicarbonate	14 mmol/l (18–22)
Glucose	5 mmol/l (2.5–6)

'Desperate Dan' needed intravenous fluids for 48 hours with hydrocortisone (cortisol) three times a day. At discharge home 10 days later, he was taking hydrocortisone 5 mg t.d.s. (20 mg/m² per day) and a small dose of fludrocortisone to prevent salt loss. The parents were given a steroid card and instructions to double or treble his steroids during intercurrent infections. They were taught to use test sticks to monitor capillary blood glucose levels when he was unwell, and regular follow-up was arranged in the outpatient clinic.

Comment

Congenital adrenal hyperplasia (CAH) is a recessively inherited group of disorders of adrenal hormone production with an incidence of 1 in 10 000. More than 90 per cent of cases are due to a specific defect of the 21-hydroxylase enzyme (Fig. 7.11). The lack of cortisol results in excessive ACTH production which stimulates the steroid pathway, producing high (up to 100 times normal) 17-OH-progesterone levels and increased testosterone levels by the same mechanism. Salt loss will occur because of the lack of mineralocorticoid, although this is clinically significant in

92 CLINICAL CASES IN PAEDIATRICS

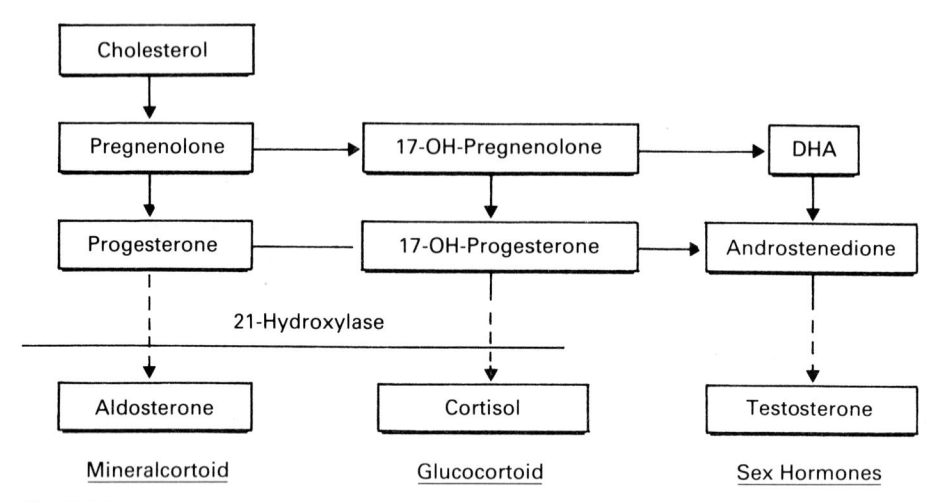

```
                        Cholesterol
                             │
                             ▼
       Pregnenolone ──→ 17-OH-Pregnenolone ──→ DHA
            │                  │                │
            ▼                  ▼                ▼
       Progesterone ── 17-OH-Progesterone ──→ Androstenedione
            │                  │                │
            ┊   21-Hydroxylase ┊                ┊
       ─────┼──────────────────┼────────────────┼─────
            ▼                  ▼                ▼
        Aldosterone         Cortisol        Testosterone

       Mineralcortoid     Glucocortoid      Sex Hormones
```

Fig. 7.11
Pathways of adrenal hormone synthesis

Table 7.6

Clinical presentation of congenital adrenal hyperplasia

Ambiguous genitalia in the female newborn, due to virilization *in utero*

Salt-losing crisis at 1–4 weeks of age (usually males since female salt losers have been recognized because of ambiguous genitalia)

Virilization in older children

---

only half the cases. The clinical presentation of CAH can thus be in three ways (Table 7.6).

Long-term management aims to produce normal growth and to minimize the risk of adrenal crises. Excessive replacement steroid will stunt growth whereas insufficient treatment will allow too much androgen production, leading to rapid growth, premature epiphyseal fusion and a very short final height. Often enthusiasm for treatment leads to too much replacement steroid, particularly during the first year of life, and stunts growth. Mineralocortocoid therapy is given to salt losers like Dan. The doses of glucocorticoid and mineralocorticoid must be optimal for satisfactory growth.

Genetic counselling should be offered to families, as there is a 1 in 4 risk of future children being affected. Antenatal diagnosis is now possible, although this presents ethical problems. Further children should have their 17-OH-progesterone levels measured at 36 hours of age so that an early diagnosis can be made. Optimal management of these children with CAH requires skill and is best left to an expert if the child's full growth potential is to be achieved.

8 Renal diseases

Urinary Tract Infection

David, who was nearly 5 years old, was seen at school for his routine medical examination. During the preceding two weeks, he had started bed wetting and complained of pain when passing urine. He had previously been fit and well; however, when questioned in detail, his mother recalled two episodes of dysuria five and seven months before which had been treated with courses of antibiotics. Sadly, no urine sample had been taken for culture.

A careful examination revealed no abnormal physical signs, and a midstream urine was collected at the clinic. David's mother was given another sterile container for collection of a second specimen at home. In order to be sure that David was not diabetic, his urine was tested for glucose. A seven-day course of co-trimoxazole was then commenced. Both urine cultures grew significant numbers of *E. coli*, fulfilling the criteria for diagnosis of urinary tract infection (Table 8.1). The doctor felt an intravenous urogram (IVU) might be indicated, so she arranged an outpatient referral. The paediatrician agreed with this and arranged follow-up. The IVU and micturating cystogram were both normal.

Comment

David had a symptomatic urinary tract infection (UTI) which develops in 1 per cent of boys and 3 per cent of girls before the age of 10 years. The relatively higher frequency of girls at older ages is shown in Table 8.2. The clinical features of UTI vary with age, and are often non-specific (Table 8.3).

There are a variety of methods for collecting 'clean' urine samples in children (clean catch, midstream urine, bag urine), and the technique of suprapubic aspiration, sometimes used in children under 18 months, is demonstrated in Fig. 8.1. Symptoms suggestive of urine infection should never be treated unless adequate samples have been obtained.

Nearly one-half of children with UTI have anatomical renal tract abnormalities, so

Table 8.1
Diagnosis of urinary tract infection

Two clean, fresh specimens of urine with a pure growth of 100 000 or more organisms/ml on culture
Any pure growth from a urine specimen taken by suprapubic aspiration of the bladder

Proteinuria and the presence or absence of pus cells are not consistently helpful

Table 8.2
Sex ratio (female : male) of urinary infections at different ages

First month of life	0.4 : 1
7–12 months	4 : 1
2–11 years	10 : 1

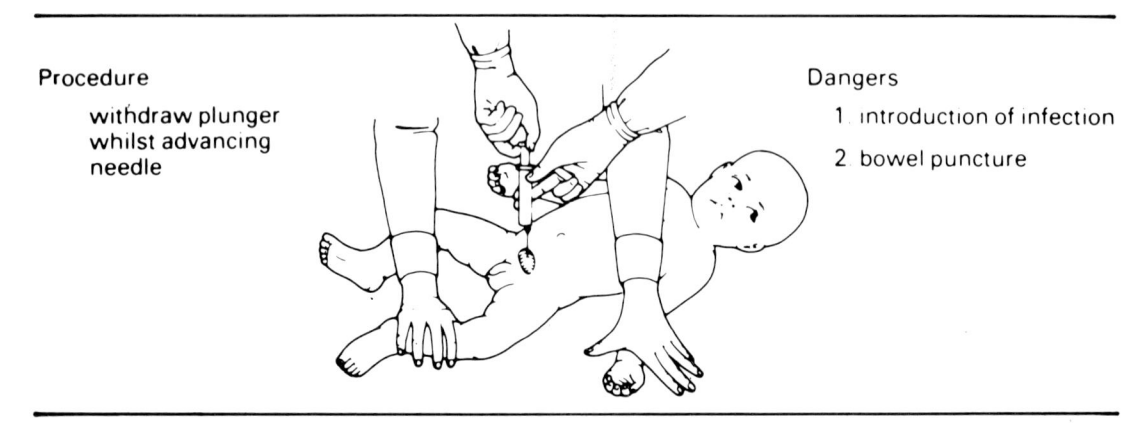

Fig. 8.1
Technique of suprapubic aspiration of urine (*From Milner AD & Hull D (1984)* Hospital Paediatrics. *Churchill Livingstone, Edinburgh, by courtesy of the publishers*)

Procedure
withdraw plunger whilst advancing needle

Dangers
1. introduction of infection
2. bowel puncture

Table 8.3
Clinical features of urinary infection

0–2 years old	Vomiting, fever, malaise Failure to thrive
2–12 years old	Fever, abdominal pain Frequency, dysuria, haematuria and enuresis Asymptomatic

thresholds for x-ray investigation, especially in boys, are much lower than in adults. Recurrent UTIs are common, as 75 per cent of children will have a reinfection within two years. David was empirically given a low dose prophylactic antibiotic for a year (trimethoprim once nightly). The urine, which was checked by his family doctor ten days later, and at three-month intervals with a dipslide, remained sterile. Further management includes advice to avoid bubble baths in girls, who have a shorter urethra than boys, and to ensure that three hours is the longest time allowed between visits to the toilet—even when busy!

The prognosis for uncomplicated urinary infections, even when recurrent, is excellent. Renal scarring and damage may result from infection if vesicoureteric reflux is also present.

Vesicoureteric Reflux

Stuart, a 5 year old was seen with a two-day history of symptoms suggestive of a urinary tract infection. Two urine cultures were taken on separate occasions and both grew a significant quantity of Proteus sensitive to trimethoprim and nitrofurantoin. Further tests were arranged after a few weeks, once his infection had been eradicated. An IVU demonstrated a dilated renal pelvis, clubbed calyces and an enlarged ureter on the left side, with no abnormalities on the right side (Fig. 8.2). The cystogram revealed bilateral reflux of urine into the ureters, severe on the left but minimal on the right side (Fig. 8.3). There was no evidence of bladder outflow obstruction from posterior urethral valves.

In view of his age, vesicoureteric reflux and infection, long-term prophylactic trimethoprim was given on a once daily basis. No further UTI occurred over the next five years.

RENAL DISEASES 95

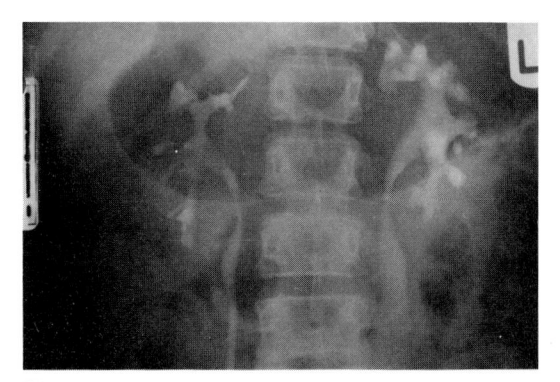

Fig. 8.2

Intravenous urogram with features suggestive of left-sided reflux

A renal isotope scan after 14 months showed normal renal growth, no scarring of the kidney and a reduction in the left-sided reflux. Five years later the scan was normal.

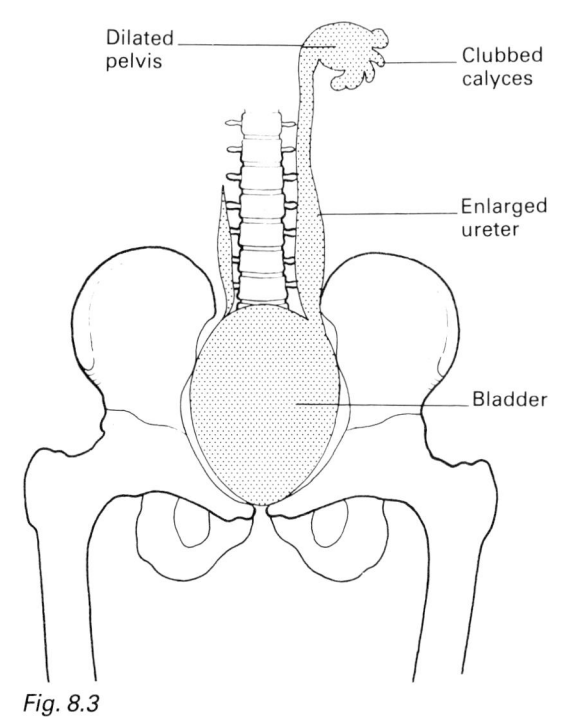

Fig. 8.3

Diagram of cystogram showing gross reflux on the left, with minimal reflux on the right side

Comment

Urine infections are common in children and by themselves do not give rise to renal scarring and permanent damage. However, the combination of infection and reflux during the first few years of life is a potent cause of such changes, which may lead to chronic renal failure (Fig. 8.4). Approximately one-third of children investigated for urine infections have coexistent reflux.

Reflux is caused by a short intramural portion of ureter leading to an incompetent vesicoureteric junction. Severity is assessed by the cystogram appearances (Table 8.4). When

Table 8.4

Classification of reflux based on cystogram findings

Grade 1	Incomplete reflux into the ureter(s), not reaching the kidney
Grade 2	Complete filling of the ureter but no dilatation of the calyces
Grade 3	Dilated calyces
Grade 4	Hydronephrosis and dilated ureter

reflux is gross, back pressure of urine allows reflux of urine within the kidney itself—intrarenal reflux. The combination of this and infection in a young child is highly likely to lead to renal scars. Thus the main significance of reflux lies in its association with infection and scarring. Some 90 per cent of children with scars have reflux. Long-term follow-up studies indicate that reflux disappears spontaneously over a period of years in all but the worst types. It is a very uncommon finding in teenagers and adults.

Management involves the prevention of urine infections and monitoring of growth and blood pressure. Because infections may

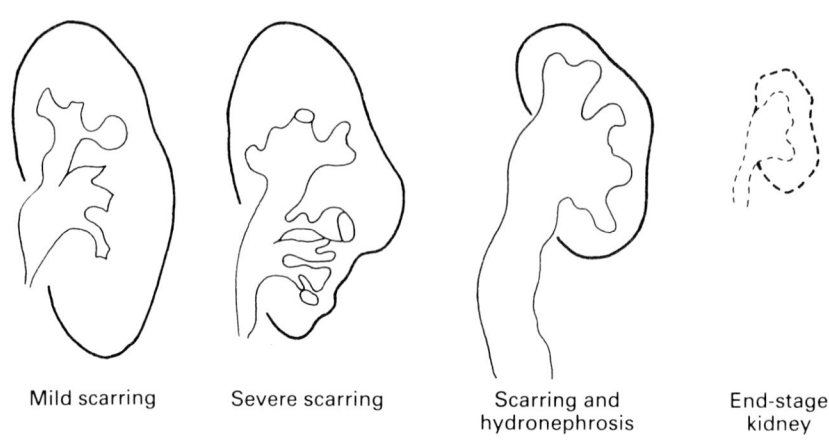

Fig. 8.4
Natural history of severe renal scarring

Mild scarring — Severe scarring — Scarring and hydronephrosis — End-stage kidney

be asymptomatic, regular urine cultures at three-month intervals are an obligatory part of the follow-up of reflux. Double voiding of urine at bedtime and long-term prophylactic antibiotics are the mainstay of treatment. The presence of reflux with sterile urine is unlikely to lead to kidney damage. Surgical reimplantation of ureters may be necessary on occasions in severe cases or if poor drug compliance makes conservative treatment impossible. It is hoped that in the future there will be a reduction in the 20–25 per cent of patients on chronic dialysis/transplant lists with end-stage kidneys from the combination of scarring and reflux.

Bed Wetting

Mandy, aged 6 years, was referred for a second opinion about her bed wetting. This had always been present, although she had been dry by day for three years. Her mother was fed up with the need to wash the sheets every day. Mandy and her 2-year-old brother Darren lived with their mother at the maternal grandparents' home, as the parents had separated two years earlier. The home was a three-bedroomed flat near the city centre, in a street with several derelict houses.

The grandmother appeared to undertake most of the care of the children and their mother had a late evening job said to involve working as a barmaid in a local hotel in the red light area of town. Mandy's mother had a social worker who was intermittently involved with the family when crises arose. The health visitor known to the family for several years found that a great deal of support was needed, especially when relations between mother and grandmother became tense.

At examination Mandy was found to be a normal 6 year old with a somewhat limited vocabulary. Her urine was checked for glucose and sent for culture. The doctor had a long discussion with Mandy and her mother about general measures to help them (see below), and arranged a further visit to the outpatient clinic after he had had time to find out more information from the family's health visitor and social worker.

Comment

Most children learn to be dry by day at 2 years and by night at 3 years. By 5 years 15 per cent of children wet their beds but this is reduced to 5 per cent by 10 years. The problem is more common in boys, especially those in lower social groups. Generally the sphincter control is poor during the night while the child is deeply asleep. Uncommon presentations of diabetes or urine infection must always be excluded. A history of continuously leaking urine will alert one to the possibility of an ectopic ureter, whereas neurological signs of a paraparesis should be easy to elicit. Bed wetting is due to an isolated delay in achieving bladder control and is often familial (like late walking or talking).

Management centres around accelerating a natural cure. Concern and time spent listening and giving encouragement will be well received. The frequency of the condition in children of a similar age should be explained and a reward system using star charts or bribery can sometimes be helpful. Drugs have been used since the Middle Ages but most have fallen into disrepute (Fig. 8.5); however, imipramine does offer temporary help and may help to restore confidence.

Thomas Phaer   Boke on Children

ON PYSSINGE IN THE BED

Take the wesande (trachea) of a cocke and plucke it, then brenne it in pouder, and use it twise or thryse a day. The stones of a hedge-hogge poudred is of the same vertue.

Fig. 8.5
Modern drug therapy for bed wetting

In this case social factors in the home will make management very difficult. When there are family tensions, marital upheavals or financial insecurity in a deprived family, inevitably compliance with treatment will be poor. Support and practical help with washing may actually be more useful than tablets or other measures. Certainly a buzzer alarm can be helpful in well motivated families, especially in children over 6 years old. The treatment of bed wetting can be rewarding, but side effects of treatment such as accidental poisoning of smaller children with tricyclic drugs should not be forgotten.

Nephrotic Syndrome

Joanne, aged 3 years, became unwell over several days. Her parents noticed her to be pale and listless with a poor appetite, and after a few days they became aware of facial swelling first thing in the morning. This had steadily worsened and a visit to see the family doctor was therefore arranged.

At examination she found generalized oedema and ascites as well as pallor. The blood pressure was 90/60 mm Hg and urine testing with a Labstix revealed heavy proteinuria but no blood or sugar. Hospital admission was therefore arranged so that further investigation and treatment could be instituted. The serum albumin was found to be 20 g/l and the serum cholesterol was high, confirming a diagnosis of nephrotic syndrome (Table 8.5).

Table 8.5
Diagnosis of the nephrotic syndrome

Oedema
Proteinuria
Hypoproteinaemia
Hypercholesterolaemia

Her serum complement level was normal and an index of protein excretion in the urine showed a highly selective pattern.

Oral prednisolone (60 mg/m^2) was started. On the fourth day of admission Joanne developed abdominal pains and became unwell. Her haematocrit had been rising from the day of admission and, since there were no features to suggest infection, it was assumed she was hypovolaemic. A salt-poor albumin infusion produced symptomatic improvement within a few hours.

Remission was induced after two weeks of steroids so that all manifestations of disease disappeared. The steroid dose was then slowly reduced and stopped after six weeks. There were three relapses during the next 18 months, which required further short courses of steroids.

Table 8.6

Comparison of the findings in acute nephritis and in nephrotic syndrome

	Acute nephritis	Nephrotic syndrome
Oedema	+	+++
Blood pressure	Raised	Normal
Urine findings:		
Protein	++	++++
Red cells	++++	Nil
White cells	++	Nil
Cellular casts	++	Nil

Comment

Nephrotic syndrome is seen in only 1 in 40 000 children, the peak incidence being between 2 and 3 years. Acute nephritis does present with mild oedema but this should be easy to distinguish from nephrotic syndrome by the presence of haematuria and hypertension (Table 8.6). About 90 per cent of nephrotic syndrome found in young children is secondary to minimal change nephropathy, which has normal histology with light microscopy but fusion of the foot processes of the glomerular basement membrane under the electron microscope. The fusion is not specific and is related to the degree of proteinuria. The cause of this nephropathy is unknown but is assumed to have an immunological basis.

In minimal change lesions, only small molecular weight proteins such as albumin or transferrin leak through the glomeruli. Therefore the urine protein excretion is 'highly selective' in these cases (Table 8.7). The pathogenesis of oedema is complex (Fig. 8.6).

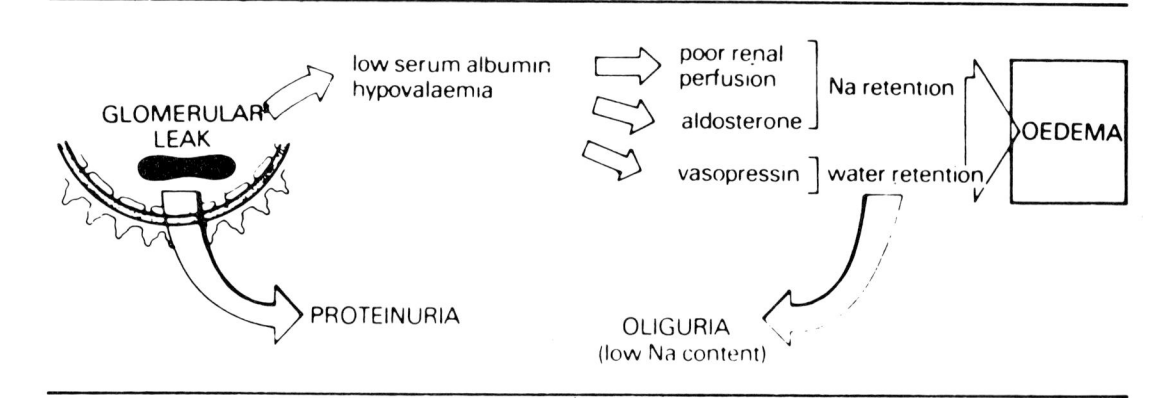

Fig. 8.6

Mechanism of glomerular protein loss (*From Milner AD & Hull D (1984)* Hospital Paediatrics. *Churchill Livingstone, Edinburgh, by courtesy of the publishers*)

Table 8.7

Protein selectivity in the nephrotic syndrome

Urine protein selectivity index is calculated by comparing the clearance of a low molecular weight protein (e.g. transferrin) with that of a high molecular weight protein (e.g. IgG)

$$\text{selectivity index} = \frac{U^a/P_a}{U^b/P_b} \frac{\text{(urine and plasma IgG concentrations)}}{\text{(urine and plasma transferrin concentrations)}}$$

high selectivity <0.1

Management includes general measures (a high protein, low salt diet) and specific drug treatment with steroids. Renal biopsy is indicated in treatment failures or atypical cases. The prognosis is excellent in the long term although there is a high relapse rate. Parents should be taught to test their child's urine for protein each day for a year after treatment, so that relapses can be treated early. On rare occasions, drugs such as cyclophosphamide may be needed to prevent multiple relapses.

Chronic Renal Failure

Sam, a 7 year old with chronic renal failure of four years' duration (Fig. 8.7), had had progressive deterioration in renal function since an episode of Henoch–Schönlein purpura. Initially he had intermittent proteinuria, but this became gradually continuous and his creatinine levels started to rise after a year, indicating that he had less than 25 per cent of normal renal function remaining. The main problems during the preceding year were growth failure, hypertension which needed treatment with propranolol and renal osteodystrophy treated with 1-α-cholecalciferol.

Sam was referred to the regional paediatric nephrologist for advice on further management. He found renal function, as assessed by glomerular filtration, to be 4 ml/1.73 m² per minute (normal 90–140), and noted the results

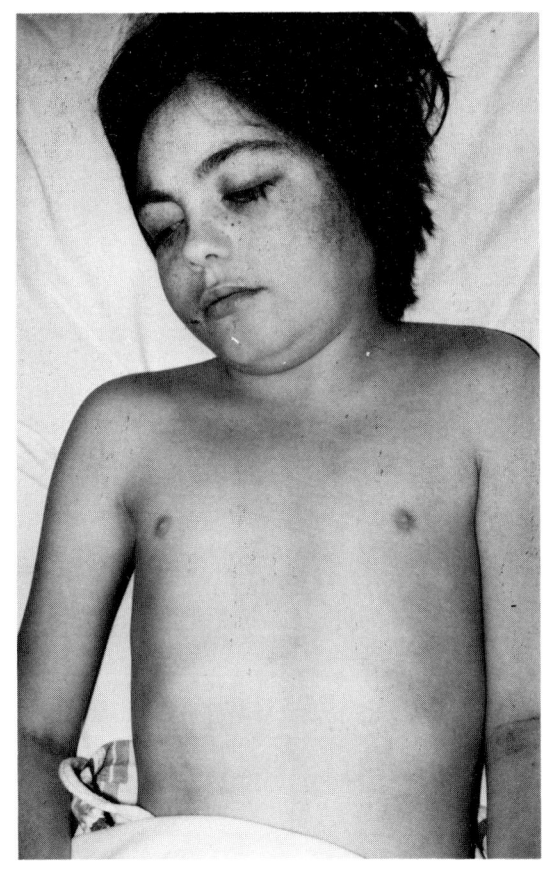

Fig. 8.7
Child with chronic renal failure

of a previous renal biopsy which showed end-stage chronic glomerulonephritis. Since there was no sudden change in Sam's condition,

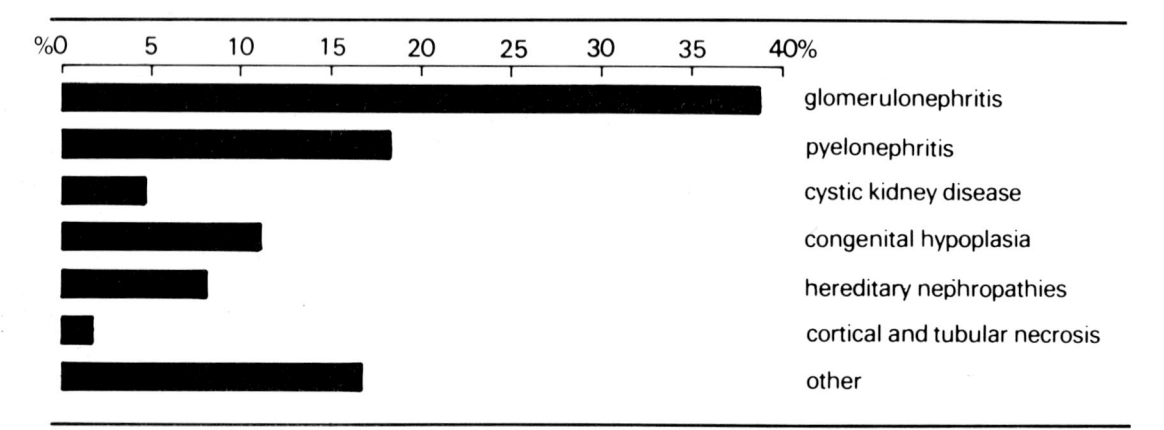

Fig. 8.8
Aetiology of chronic renal failure (*From Milner AD & Hull D (1984)* Hospital Paediatrics. *Churchill Livingstone, Edinburgh, by courtesy of the publishers*)

there was time for full assessment of the family unit by the renal dialysis team, which included a nurse, social worker, dietitian, teacher and child psychiatrist. A unanimous decision to pursue a plan of haemodialysis, followed by transplantation when possible, was suggested as the parents were keen for active treatment and Sam was felt likely to cope with such intensive treatment better than most.

An arteriovenous fistula was inserted into his left arm and twice-weekly haemodialysis was carried out whilst he was awaiting a kidney. Fortunately, after seven months one became available and he received a transplant. Steroids and azathioprine were given to prevent rejection, and discharge home was allowed after two weeks. In spite of the hospital visits and blood tests which were still needed, his quality of life was improved.

Comment

A hundred children a year develop chronic renal failure, with chronic glomerulonephritis and pyelonephritis (reflux nephropathy) accounting for more than half the cases (Fig. 8.8). The kidney has several physiological roles, which are all disturbed in chronic renal failure (Fig. 8.9). Homoeostasis is there-

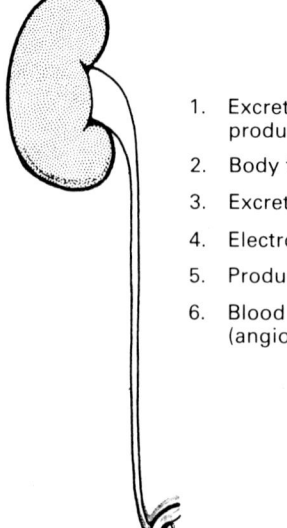

1. Excretion of protein breakdown products (urea, creatinine, etc.)
2. Body fluid homoeostasis
3. Excretion of H^+
4. Electrolyte homoeostasis
5. Production of erythropoietin
6. Blood pressure homoeostasis (angiotensin-renin system)

Fig. 8.9
Functions of kidneys

Table 8.8
Conservative management of chronic renal failure

Encourage maximal renal function with a high fluid intake
Low protein diet
Treatment of hypertension
Treatment of renal osteodystrophy
Prompt treatment of urinary infection

fore deranged in children with chronic renal failure in a similar way to adults. The effect on growth is usually very marked indeed.

Conservative management by diet and drugs is indicated for milder cases (Table 8.8). Treatment of anaemia by transfusion is generally not needed, as children tolerate moderate anaemia well. For severely affected children, home haemodialysis offers a three-year survival of 90 per cent, and haemodialysis in hospital 80 per cent. Technical problems can arise from difficulties of vascular access from a Silastic shunt or arteriovenous fistula, and families need prolonged training in the use of the equiment at home. Continuous ambulatory peritoneal dialysis now offers an alternative form of treatment.

In the best centres one-year survival is 70 per cent for the transplanted kidney and 92 per cent for the child. A return to normal life will usually be possible after three months. As with any chronic disease in children, especially if the treatment is demanding, emotional and social factors in the family are just as important as medical ones in determining the final outcome.

9 Infectious diseases

Malaria

Geeta, the 11-year-old daughter of Indian parents, presented with a three-week history of fever, sweats and rigors. Her appetite had been poor and she complained of severe headache associated with nausea and vomiting. Geeta was born in the UK, and had visited Bombay with her parents ten weeks earlier. A seven-day course of ampicillin from her family doctor had not improved her symptoms.

She looked unwell and had a temperature of 39°C with cold sores around her mouth. Her liver was tender but not enlarged, and there was an enlarged spleen. A routine blood count was normal except for a mild anaemia (Hb 9.8 g/dl). In view of the recent foreign travel, malaria was suspected. The typical pattern of fever often is not present early in the disease, and may not arise at all in younger children (Fig. 9.1).

The haematologist was requested to search specifically for malarial parasites on the blood film. A thin film revealed that nearly 1 per cent of the red cells were parasitized by ring trophozoites, typical of *Plasmodium vivax* (Fig. 9.2). It is unusual to have many more red cells involved in vivax malaria, and this can make the diagnosis difficult. With low levels of infection, thick films showing lysed erythrocytes may help. Mixed infections are sometimes seen with more than one malarial parasite.

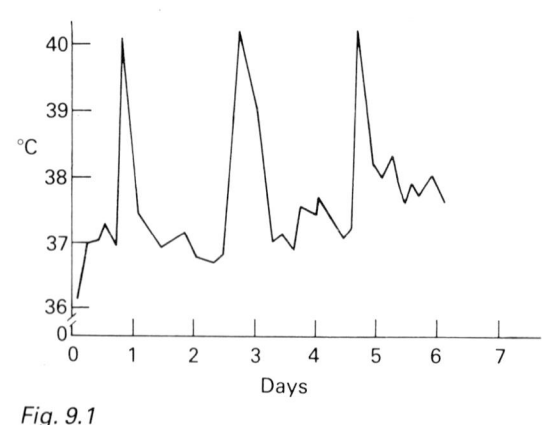

Fig. 9.1

Temperature chart in *Plasmodium vivax* infection

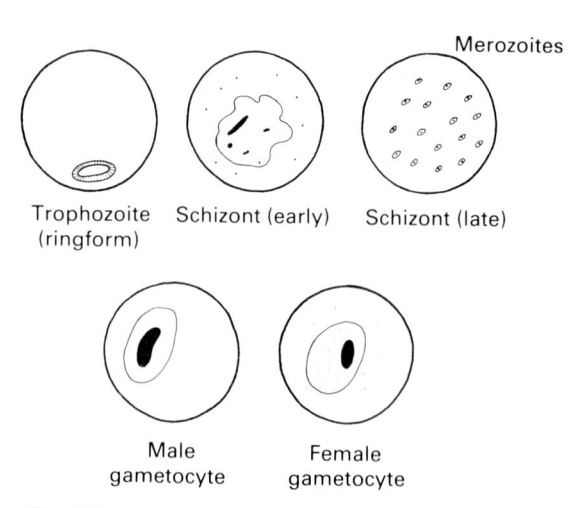

Fig. 9.2

Appearance of malarial parasites in *Plasmodium vivax* infection

Comment

There are about 1600 diagnosed cases of malaria in the UK each year. A diagnosis of malaria should always be considered in children visiting or coming from a malaria area, even if prophylactic drugs have been taken, because compliance may be poor. Geeta was in fact visiting an area without chloroquine resistance, which is now present in parts of Central/South America, Asia and Africa (Fig. 9.3). Fortunately, benign tertian malaria (*P. vivax*) rarely gives rise to complications, but the greater parasitization with malignant tertian malaria due to *P. falciparum* (up to 20 per cent of red cells) can cause major illness and death.

Drug resistance, partial immunity and poor compliance render the treatment of malaria a field for the expert, but advice is readily available from a number of centres in England and Scotland. Geeta was in fact treated with chloroquine to eradicate the infection, followed up by primaquine to prevent relapse which can occur up to two years later. Her symptoms rapidly improved and advice was given about chemoprophylaxis for future travel abroad.

Chickenpox

Mrs E was admitted to hospital at 39 weeks' gestation with a six-day history of a rash typical of chickenpox. A few hours after admission she went into spontaneous labour and delivered a normal female baby who was in good condition at birth. Samantha had no stigmata of chickenpox. Nevertheless, it was decided to administer a dose of intramuscular zoster immunoglobulin immediately after delivery as prophylaxis against neonatal chickenpox, since this disease has a significant mortality. Mother and daughter were barrier nursed for a week, by which time the mother's rash had disappeared. They were discharged home and the parents were given instructions

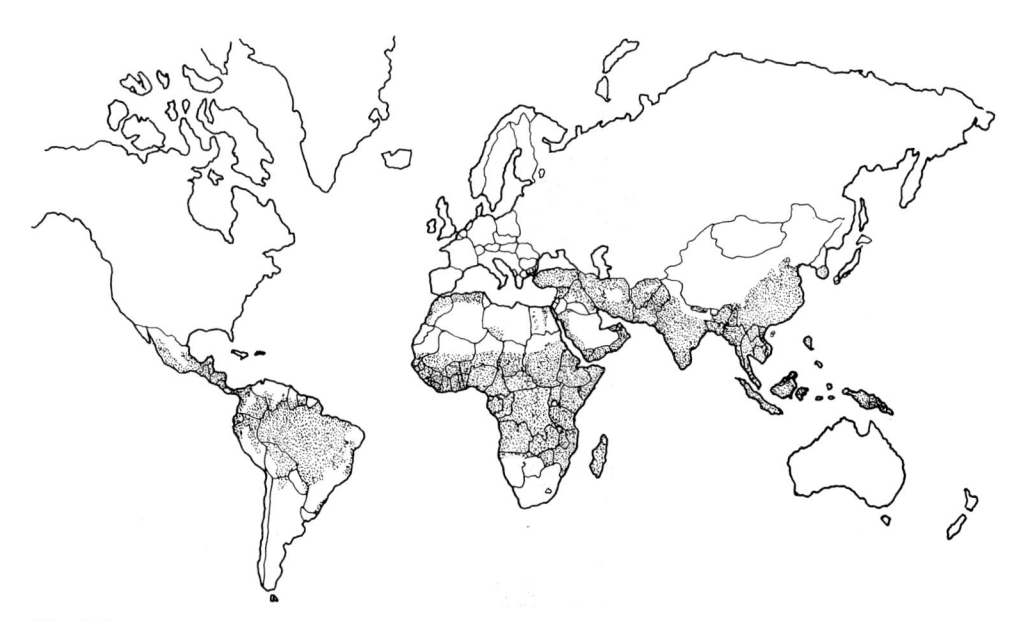

Fig. 9.3
World map of malaria areas

to bring Samantha back to hospital if any rash developed over the next two weeks.

Comment

Chickenpox is a common, relatively minor disease of childhood. The first sign of illness is usually the rash, but a prodromal period of fever, headache, sore throat and malaise may be the initial presenting features in adults. The typical centripetal distribution of the rash, an enanthem (palate and fauces) and the rash itself, which evolves through four stages—macule, papule, vesicle and pustule—enables confident diagnosis to be made in nearly all cases. Smallpox has now been eradicated world wide, so this disease no longer causes diagnostic problems.

Complications of the disease (Table 9.1) are

Table 9.1

Complications of chickenpox

Secondary bacterial infections of the rash
Chickenpox pneumonia
Haemorrhagic chickenpox
Encephalitis (especially involving the cerebellum)

rare in children, apart from secondary bacterial infection of the rash due to scratching. Certain children are considered at risk from chickenpox and are likely to develop serious or life-threatening disease (Table 9.2).

Most women of childbearing age have had chickenpox, but the disease can cause fetal skin scarring if contracted early in pregnancy. The virus can cross the placenta, so if the mother had chickenpox at the end of the pregnancy, the infant may be born with the disease or develop it within the first three weeks of life. The mortality from neonatal chickenpox

Table 9.2

Those at risk of developing severe chickenpox

The fetus
Newborn infants
Immunosuppressed children:
    With malignant disease, especially leukaemia
    Under treatment with cytoxic drugs and/or radiotherapy
    On steroids

is high when the mother develops a rash within three days of delivery. If the rash has been present longer than this, the neonatal illness is usually mild because maternal IgG antibody will have been produced in sufficient quantity to cross the placenta and partially protect the infant. Evidence suggests that zoster immunoglobulin given at birth protects the infant when the mother has chickenpox. In the case of invasive neonatal chickenpox, acyclovir will be indicated, as this is effective against the herpes zoster virus and is thought to have few side effects.

Measles

Daniel, 20 months old, was brought up to his doctor's surgery with a two-day illness. He had been miserable with a fever, cough and runny nose. His eyes were sticky and his left lower eyelid was swollen. Daniel had three siblings and his mother was unmarried. There had been housing and financial problems during the last year, but the social worker felt the home situation was now more stable.

On examination he was extremely miserable, with pyrexia (temperature 38.3°C), a runny nose, hacking cough and bilateral conjunctivitis. Inside his mouth, small white spots were seen on the reddened buccal mucosa opposite the molar teeth. No skin rash was present but a confident diagnosis of measles was made on the basis of the history, signs of a respiratory infection and the presence of these Koplik spots which appear a day or so before the rash. He was sent home to bed and his mother was advised to give him regular paracetamol elixir and plenty of fluids.

Two days later the health visitor requested a home visit from the doctor because Daniel had a temperature of 40°C and was vomiting. A typical measles rash with confluent maculopapular blotches most marked on his face and upper trunk was present. Both eardrums were red and bulging, confirming the presence of otitis media, which was treated with ampicillin (first dose intramuscularly).

Comment

The incidence of complications of this disease is still high (Table 9.3). The rare complication

Table 9.3

Complications of measles

Pneumonia	incidence 1 in 25
Otitis media	incidence 1 in 30
Encephalitis	incidence 1 in 1000
Subacute sclerosing panencephalitis (up to 10 years later)	incidence 1 in 100 000
In developing countries, measles may be complicated by diarrhoea, malnutrition and cancrum oris, and is often fatal	

of encephalitis has a 20 per cent mortality, and subacute sclerosing panencephalitis (SSPE) which can develop years later is nearly always fatal.

Immunization was introduced in 1963 in the USA and in 1968 in the UK, using a live attenuated virus vaccine. It is given at about 15 months, but currently only 55 per cent of children receive immunization in the UK. With high immunization rates the disease could be eradicated, and encephalitis and SSPE would disappear (Fig. 9.4). There are very few contraindications to immunization. Mild pyrexia, sometimes with a rash, is commonly seen about seven to ten days afterwards.

Immunization is especially important for children in institutions, those with congenital heart disease or cystic fibrosis, and in children in developing countries where morbidity and mortality are so much greater. An outbreak of measles in a family or hospital can be prevented by active immunization if given within three days of contact, as the incubation period of vaccine measles (ten days) is several days shorter than natural measles (13 days). In children with contraindications to active immunizations (for example, immunosuppressed children), passive immunity may be induced for a month by giving pooled gammaglobulin by intramuscular injection.

Congenital Rubella

Justin was born at 38 weeks' gestation to a West Indian mother, following a pregnancy that had been normal except for a mild febrile illness without any detectable rash at about 12 weeks' gestation. His birth weight was 1.94 kg (small for dates). When he was 4 hours old, a generalized petechial rash appeared, and hepatosplenomegaly was discovered. An infection screen failed to grow any bacterial pathogens but the blood count demonstrated thrombocytopenia with a platelet count of $30 \times 10^9/l$. Examination of the eyes revealed an absent light reflex from the left pupil when an ophthalmoscope was shone in the eyes from 10 cm away. The eye was small and the fundus could not be visualized because of a dense cataract. The left eye appeared normal,

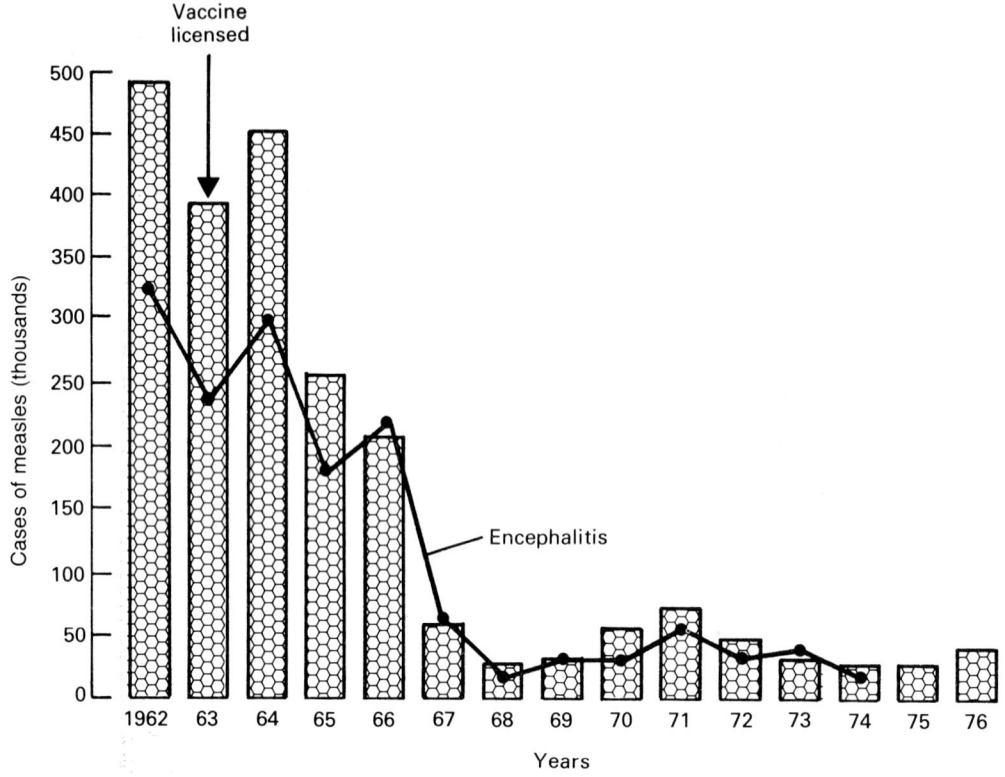

Fig. 9.4
Reduction in incidence of measles encephalitis and SSPE in USA

but the fundus was dotted with fine deposits of pigment (salt and pepper retinopathy).

The possibility of congenital infection was considered, and 'TORCH' (toxoplasmosis, rubella, cytomegalovirus and herpes) antibodies were measured in the mother and infant. Rubella-specific IgM was isolated from Justin, confirming a diagnosis of congenital rubella infection. Rubella-specific IgG was also present but not significant because it readily crosses the placenta and usually represents maternal antibody. Rubella virus was subsequently isolated from a nasopharyngeal aspirate and from the urine.

In view of the diagnosis, Justin's hearing was tested at 2 weeks in an auditory response cradle, which assesses the infant's response to sound stimuli. Responses measured are head turn, body activity, startle and respiratory pattern. There was no response to any sound on several occasions, so profound deafness was thought to be present. At 5 months a 70 decibel hearing loss indicated profound deafness and a hearing aid fitted.

From birth, Justin's rate of growth was slow and he remained below the 3rd percentile for height and weight. His hepatosplenomegaly persisted for several weeks before finally disappearing.

Comment

Rubella is generally a trivial infection of childhood. By the age of 18 years, three-quarters of the population of most countries will have had the infection. A history of previous clinical infection is unreliable because many viruses produce rubelliform rashes, and many infections are asymptomatic. A maternal rubella infection during the early stages of pregnancy produces fetal damage and evidence of congenital infection in up to 60 per cent of cases, depending on the gestation of the pregnancy at the time of exposure to rubella virus (Fig. 9.5).

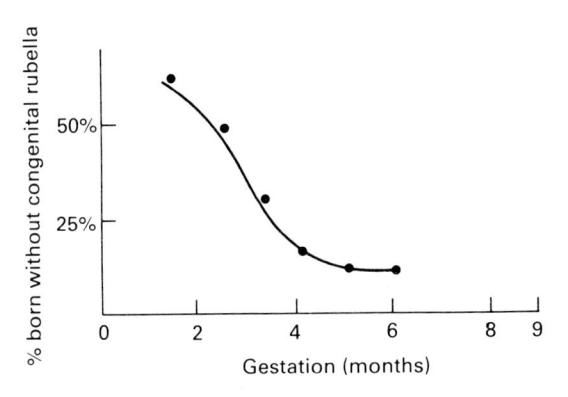

Fig. 9.5
Risk of congenital rubella following proven maternal infection

Manifestations of congenital rubella are numerous (Fig. 9.6), most causing permanent damage and handicap but some are temporary phenomena (Table 9.4). Cardiac defects are quite common, with persistent ductus arteriosus being the most frequent. The infant with congenital rubella may excrete rubella virus for up to a year, and the virus has been isolated from the lens of the eye several years later. Such infants are extremely infectious to others, and the parents should be warned.

Prevention of congenital rubella involves termination of pregnancy in proven cases and passive immunoprophylaxis with pooled gammaglobulin after known exposure of susceptible women. Immunization in the UK has been offered to early teenage schoolgirls but the uptake still needs to be improved if congenital rubella is to be eradicated. The US scheme is to immunize all infants, boys and girls, against rubella, with the aim of eradicating the illness completely.

Table 9.4
Temporary features of congenital rubella

Thrombocytopenia with purpura
Neonatal hepatitis with jaundice and hepatosplenomegaly
Osteitis with irregular metaphyseal mineralization

Acute Osteomyelitis

Sidney, a 9 year old, developed severe pain in his right knee, which started two days before he was seen by his doctor. He had not slept well because of the pain and had been febrile with a poor appetite. There was no history of bone or joint disease in the past. However, on further questioning there was a history of trauma dating from a week before when Sidney had been kicked in the leg by his sister's horse.

When examined he was febrile with a temperature of 39°C, and the skin above his right knee was hot to touch. There was a small area of exquisite tenderness over the lateral femur about 1–2 cm above the knee. Knee joint movements were painful but there was no swelling of the joint itself.

Hospital admission was arranged. The initial blood count findings were suggestive of acute infection, and serial blood cultures grew *Staphylococcus aureus* from two out of

MANIFESTATIONS OF CONGENITAL RUBELLA
(Small - for - dates. Failure to thrive)

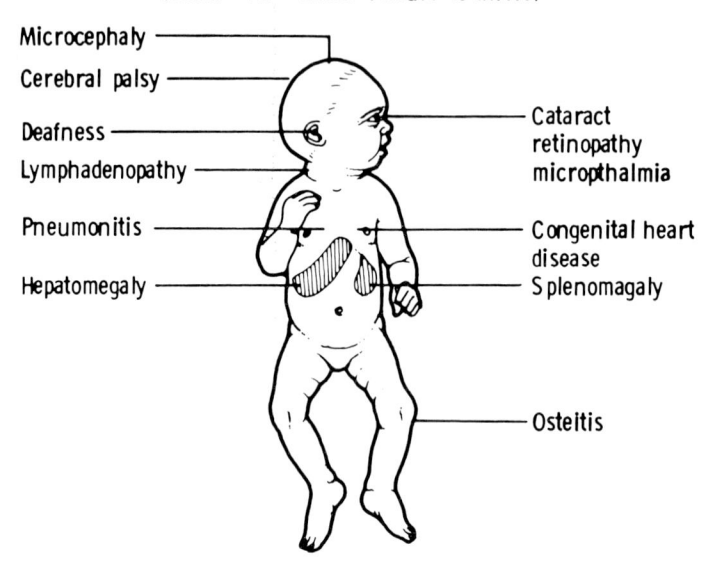

- Microcephaly
- Cerebral palsy
- Deafness
- Lymphadenopathy
- Pneumonitis
- Hepatomegaly
- Cataract, retinopathy, micropthalmia
- Congenital heart disease
- Splenomagaly
- Osteitis

Fig. 9.6
Features of congenital rubella

three sets of bottles. X-rays of the femur and knee joint were normal.

Treatment was started with ampicillin and flucloxacillin in high dosage before the culture results were returned. An orthopaedic surgeon reviewed Sidney 48 hours after admission and felt that operative treatment was unnecessary, as he appeared to be responding to treatment.

Comment

Acute osteomyelitis occurs in the newborn, but is more commonly found between the ages of 5 and 15 years. Long bones, particularly the metaphyses of the femur and tibia, are the most frequent sites of infection. A history of minor trauma is quite frequent and possibly this predisposes to infection. Open wounds from trauma or surgery can of course lead to contiguous infection, but most cases are secondary to haematogenous spread. Many are caused by *Staphylococcus aureus* although *Streptococcus pyogenes*, *Haemophilus influenzae* and salmonellae can occasionally infect bone. X-ray changes take at least ten days to develop but a radioisotope scan will show increased local uptake at an earlier stage. The diagnosis, however, is a clinical one.

Treatment involves high dose antibiotics, with initial therapy covering staphylococcal infection. Once blood culture results and sensitivities are available, antibiotic therapy can be adjusted. Generally two antibiotics are used for staphylococcal infection; e.g. flucloxacillin and fusidic acid. Complications such as chronic osteomyelitis are now uncommon with early diagnosis and treatment. Orthopaedic advice should always be sought, as subperiosteal pus or necrotic bone may need removing. Antibiotics are discontinued after six weeks and full recovery is usual.

10 Accidents and trauma

Burns

Phillip was an 8-year-old boy, who was previously fit and healthy. One evening after school he was helping his older brother to burn a pile of rubbish in their back garden. The rubbish was damp and they had difficulty in getting it to burn. Phillip poured a can of petrol over the pile, but at the same time spilt some over his trousers—as the fire was lit, so his trousers were set alight. His mother managed to put out the flames and pulled his charred clothes away.

When he arrived in hospital, he was

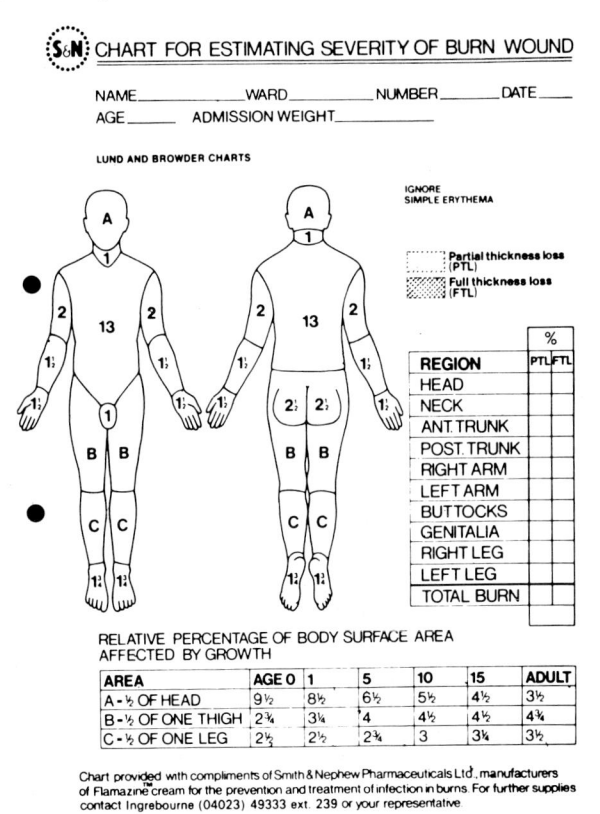

Fig. 10.1

Chart for the calculation of severity of burns
(*Supplied by Smith and Nephew Pharmaceuticals Ltd*)

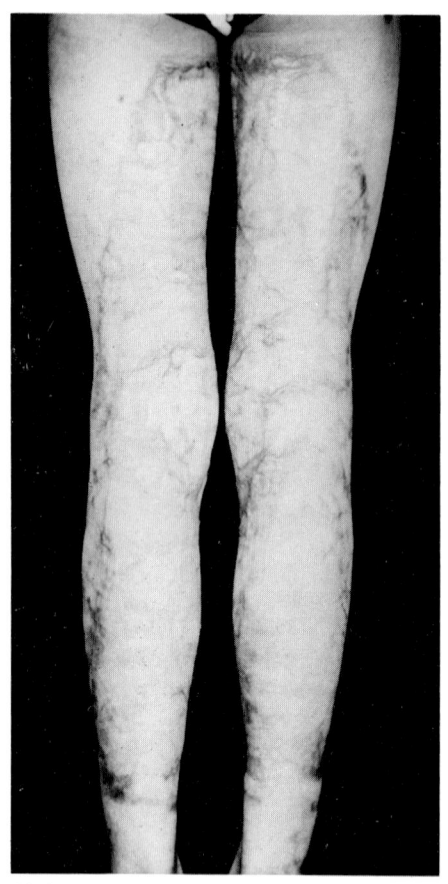

Fig. 10.2
Severe scarring following burns

screaming with pain. He had extensive blistering of most of the skin of both legs. Fortunately his trunk and arms were spared, but his hair was singed. Burns are very painful and strong analgesia is required—Phillip was given an injection of heroin immediately.

The extent of his burns was calculated from a chart which estimates the relative surface area of different parts of the body (Fig. 10.1). Note that this varies according to the age of the child. Phillip had burns which involved about 30 per cent of his body.

This is an indication for intravenous therapy, since large amounts of plasma are lost from burnt surfaces. He was given plasma transfusions and IV fluids for 24 hours after admission and was nursed in a paediatric intensive care unit, where frequent and accurate observations could be made. Management of severe burns requires meticulous observation of fluid balance, based on measurements of pulse rate, blood pressure, urine output and blood biochemical and haematocrit estimations. The first 48 hours are crucial—treatment is aimed at correcting fluid loss rather than attending to the burns themselves.

Phillip made a reasonable recovery and 48 hours later was transferred to a burns unit. Over the next month he had four separate operations to remove areas of dead, sloughed skin and to apply grafts where full-thickness burns had occurred. He now has severe scarring of both legs (Fig. 10.2).

Comment

Death from burns is the third commonest cause of accidental death in children, resulting in about 200 deaths each year in Great Britain. Of these, nearly two-thirds occur before the age of 5 years and the same proportion take place within the home. Unlike other accidents, burns are much more common in girls (perhaps because of the inflammable nature of dresses and nightdresses). Toddlers may receive burns after tipping saucepans of boiling water off cookers or pulling a kettle off a work top. Burns involving more than 70 per

Table 10.1

Immediate action in severe burns

Relieve pain with strong analgesic
Ensure an adequate airway when mouth or pharynx involved
Assess extent of burns
Set up an IV infusion and give plasma

cent of the body are rarely compatible with survival. The immediate management of a burnt child is shown in Table 10.1.

The emphasis should be on the prevention of burns by improved education. For every child fatally burned there are many who are disabled, disfigured or frightened.

Non-accidental Injury

Karen was brought up to the accident and emergency department at 8 weeks of age by her maternal grandmother who had noticed some bleeding from the baby's mouth. The casualty officer noticed a torn frenulum of the upper lip, several small facial bruises and a slight subconjunctival haemorrhage. He was not happy about the explanation for these injuries from the parents, who arrived shortly afterwards. The infant and family were seen by a paediatrician who noted that the mother was 18 and the father 21, and that they had lived together for a year with an apparently stable relationship. The social worker knew the family well because the father was unemployed and there were numerous housing and financial problems. Further questioning revealed that Karen cried a great deal during the day and that the explanation for the injuries was that they were self-inflicted during a temper tantrum.

Two investigations were carried out: a skeletal survey (looking for recent or old fractures) and coagulation studies. Karen was voluntarily admitted to hospital. The consultant paediatrician, senior social worker and the police were informed and arrangements were made to photograph the injuries. A skull x-ray showed a large linear fracture of the right parietal region, but fortunately there were no signs of intracerebral bleeding and there were no long-term sequelae.

Comment

Non-accidental injury (NAI) forms one end of the spectrum of child abuse and neglect (Table 10.2). It is estimated that NAI may be responsible for 25 per cent of fractures in infants aged under 2 years, and that its incidence is 4500 cases per year in the UK. The

Table 10.2

Child abuse and neglect

Non-accidental injury
Failure to thrive
Emotional deprivation
Sexual abuse
Deliberate poisoning
Invention of symptoms (Munchausen's syndrome by proxy)

Table 10.3

Common findings in families of non-accidental injury children

Young parents
Limited mothering skills
Emotional immaturity
Puerperal depression
Socioeconomic deprivation
Parents in care as children
Violent father
Heavy drinking

idea of causing deliberate injury to an infant or child is so repugnant that it is easy to assume that the parents are mentally ill. This is not often the case, but there are common features in such families (Table 10.3). Injuries may be inflicted by shaking or squeezing (Fig. 10.3), which leave fingertip bruises on the trunk and produce intracranial or

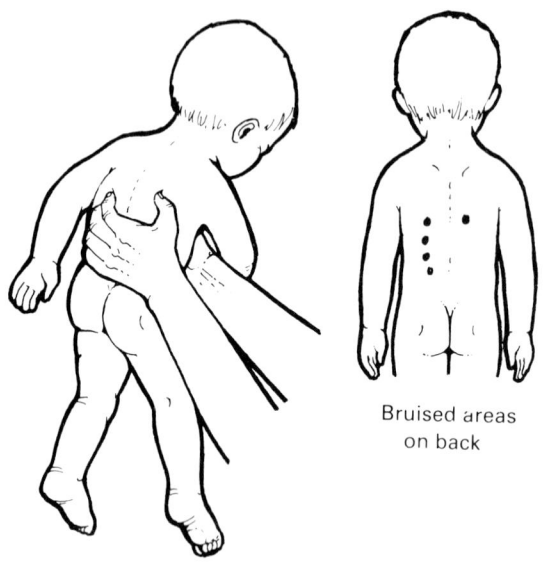

Fig. 10.3
Mechanism of bruising in non-accidental injury

Bruised areas on back

retinal haemorrhage. Burns from cigarettes or hot water are also inflicted on young children.

When non-accidental injury is suspected by a health visitor, social worker or doctor *the child must be protected against further injury* by removal to a place of safety, which may be a police station, hospital or social services home. A place of safety order, valid for four weeks, can be obtained whilst investigations are being undertaken and a case conference arranged. At this meeting of social workers, health visitors, police, doctors and other interested parties, decisions will be taken on future management of the child and family, with the interest of the child at the forefront of such plans.

In this case Karen's 2-year-old sister also had x-ray evidence of previous non-accidental injury, so a care order was obtained from the juvenile court, as it was felt by everyone that the risk to Karen was too great for her to stay with her parents. Both children were then fostered.

Near-drowning

Patrick, a 10 year old who was a keen fisherman, unfortunately tripped and fell into the river while attempting to land his catch. The recent heavy rainfall had made the currents more rapid than usual so he was swept downstream. He was rescued by a fellow angler who brought him ashore.

Fortunately another member of the local fishing club who was nearby was familiar with first aid procedures. He found Patrick unconscious and cyanosed so commenced resuscitation using mouth to mouth breathing (Fig. 10.4), with the child's head extended and his nostrils occluded. He ventilated the child at about 20 breaths per minute, but after a minute he paused to feel the pulse, which appeared absent. External cardiac massage was given by a helper following careful instruction (Fig. 10.5). A rate of 100 per minute was used without interruptions for mouth to mouth ventilation.

On arrival in the intensive care unit of the local hospital, Patrick was breathing spontaneously but needed 50% oxygen to maintain a reasonable colour. He was rousable but very

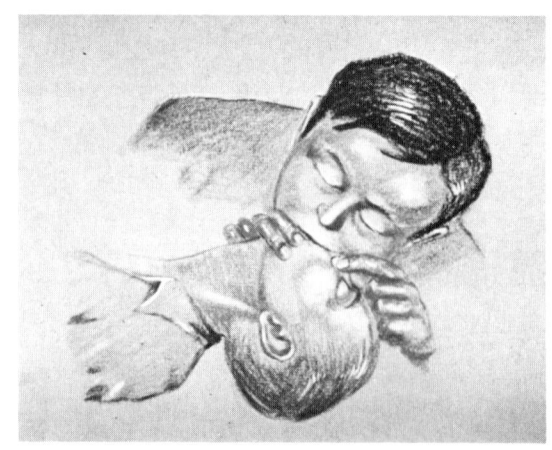

Fig. 10.4
Mouth to mouth resuscitation

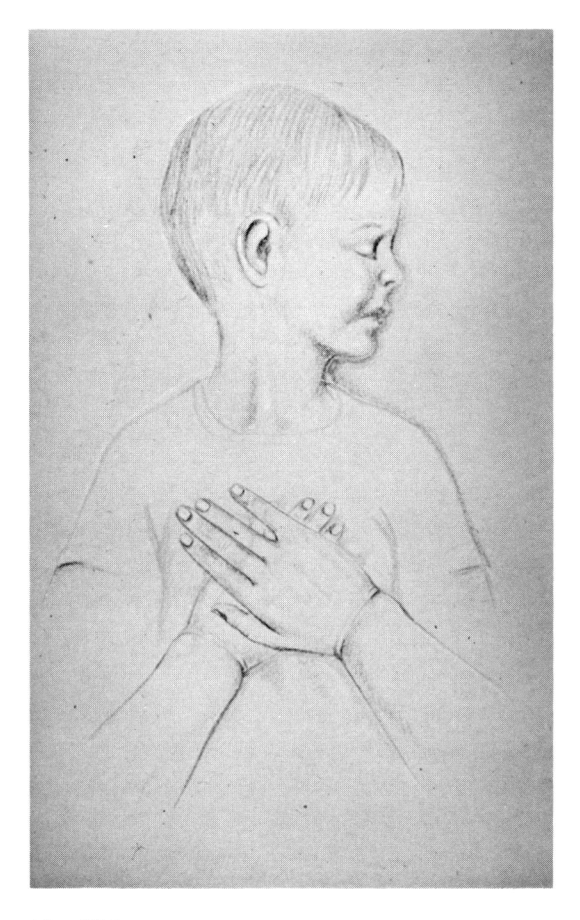

Fig. 10.5
Cardiac massage

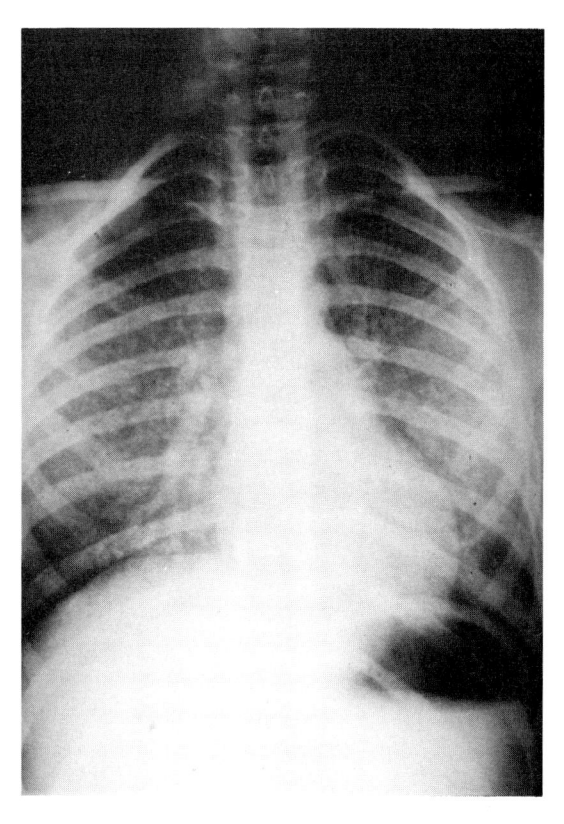

Fig. 10.6
Chest x-ray indicating pulmonary oedema

confused and unable to respond to direct questions. Coarse crackles were audible over both lung fields and his rectal temperature was 34°C. A chest x-ray showed moderate pulmonary oedema (Fig. 10.6), and arterial blood gases a picture of hypoxia and respiratory failure.

Management included the following measures: (1) mechanical ventilation using positive end-expiratory pressure (PEEP), (2) intravenous fluids restricted to one-third requirements, (3) warming blankets and (4) sedation.

Comment

There are about 300 deaths each year from drowning in the UK. Clearly the number of deaths in a country will vary with the extent of the coastline and area of inshore water, lakes and rivers.

The effects of submersion in water depend on the temperature of the water, its state of cleanliness and the age of the child. Cold water triggers the diving reflex which shuts down the peripheral circulation and also produces a bradycardia. This vestigial reflex, present in children, enables mammals to remain submerged for up to 30 minutes. Cardiac output can therefore be maintained during drowning for more than ten minutes following submersion. Recovery has been documented after 40 minutes of submersion, so resuscitation should be instituted in apparently hopeless cases. The young child will be more susceptible than the older child to hypothermia as his surface area to weight ratio will be greater. Sudden immersion in very cold water can lead to ventricular fibrillation, but more commonly loss of consciousness takes place with subsequent drowning. Hypothermia can protect the brain against asphyxial damage, and this is also responsible for the prolonged survival following circulatory arrest.

The contrasting pictures of salt and fresh water drowning have been emphasized in the past but are of little practical importance. It should be remembered that secondary drowning due to pulmonary oedema may ensue up to three days after the initial episode. This has a high mortality and should be diagnosed and treated early. In the critically ill child the advice and help of experienced anaesthetists or naval specialists with an interest in the field may prove essential, as there is good evidence that aggressive management reduces mortality as well as the risk of permanent brain damage.

Accidental Poisoning

Stephen was seen in the accident and emergency department at 3 years of age, after swallowing a number of adult aspirin tablets. His mother was not sure how many tablets had been in the bottle, and said he could have swallowed them up to six hours ago but she had not noticed the bottle at first. During the last year Stephen had been seen twice with accidental poisoning, once after eating a month's supply of contraceptive pills, and the other occasion after taking ten diazepam (Valium) tablets. There were three other children in the family, and the husband worked as a long distance lorry driver. Carl, Stephen's 2-year-old brother had had several admissions for failure to thrive without any medical cause being found, and it was noted that he always gained weight during his hospital stays.

Baseline salicylate levels were taken and repeated six hours later. They showed levels of 3 mmol/l (42 mg/100 ml) and 3.5 mmol/l (49 mg/100 ml) respectively, so no specific treatment was given (Fig. 10.7). Because this was the third episode of accidental poisoning, a social worker was asked to look into the family circumstances in more detail. Further information was obtained from the health

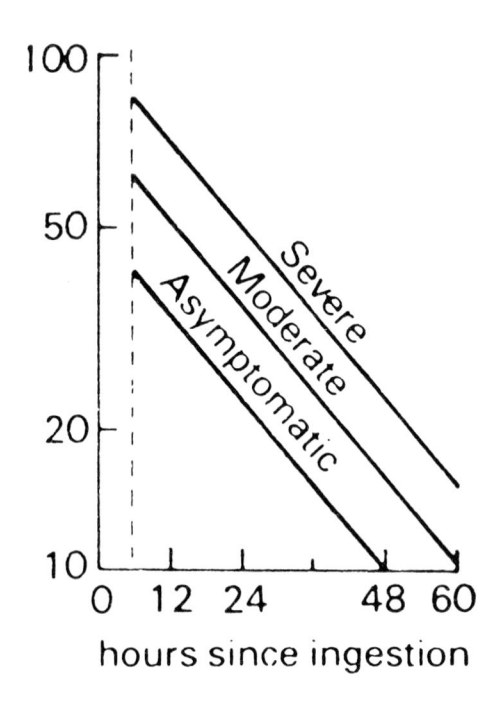

Fig. 10.7

Assessment of severity of salicylate poisoning (levels in mg per 100 ml) (*From Milner AD & Hull D (1984)* Hospital Paediatrics. *Churchill Livingstone, Edinburgh, by courtesy of the publishers*)

visitor and from previous reports during Carl's hospital admissions. It was felt that the mother had difficulty coping with four children and there was little support from her husband or family. She generally let the children 'get on by themselves' without much in the way of supervision.

A day nursery place was arranged for Stephen so that he could attend each morning during the week. Further advice was given on keeping drugs and toxic household products out of reach or in locked cupboards.

Comment

There are about 40 deaths a year from accidental poisoning, which make up only a small proportion of all children's deaths from accidents (Fig. 10.8). Nevertheless, 16 000 children are admitted to hospital each year and 40 000 attend accident and emergency departments as a result of accidental ingestion. The mean age of these children is around 3 years (Fig. 10.9) and, surprisingly, the incidence is equal for boys and girls under 5 years old; most other accidents are more common in boys.

A normal toddler explores his environment and learns from experience. Most poisoning occurs at a stage of the child's development when he is inquisitive and tends to climb, taste, bite and explore around himself. Prevention of accidents of all types involves the use of physical safeguards such as fireguards, gates at the top of stairs, and the use of child-resistant containers for drugs. The last have reduced the incidence of drug poisoning by 80 per cent.

Salicylate poisoning can be fatal, and the management depends on blood levels in relation to the time since ingestion (Table 10.4). With moderate or severe poisoning a dextrose–saline infusion with alkaline diuresis is employed, with careful monitoring of blood sugars to detect hypoglycaemia.

Occasionally dialysis may be needed if renal failure develops, and an exchange blood transfusion has been advocated in the severest cases. Other types of poisoning with

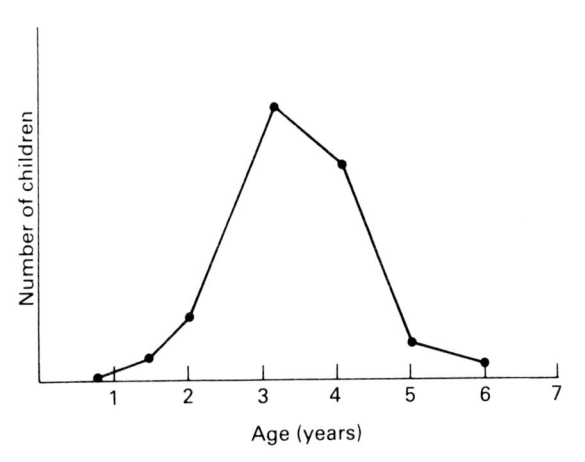

Fig. 10.9
Age distribution of children admitted to hospital with accidental poisoning

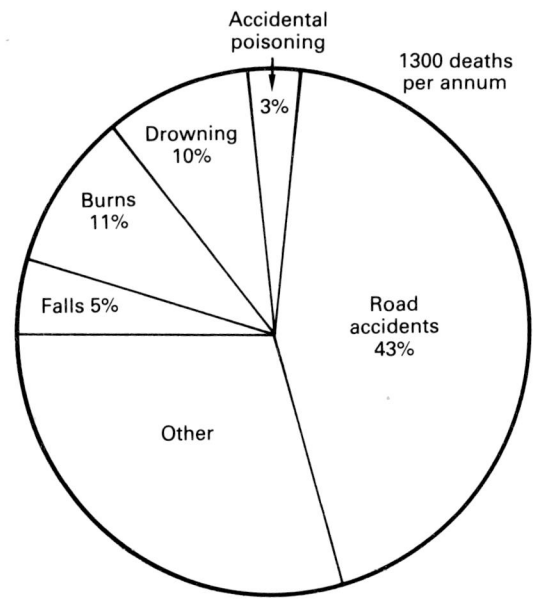

Fig. 10.8
Accidental deaths in children 0 to 14 years

Table 10.4

Treatment of salicylate poisoning

Salicylate level (4–6 hours after ingestion)	Treatment
Less than 45 mg/dl (asymptomatic)	None
45–65 mg/dl (mild)	Encourage a high fluid intake (IV if necessary)
Above 65 mg/dl (moderate or severe)	Intravenous fluids, forced alkaline diuresis

sedatives and sleeping tablets are common, but no specific treatment is needed. Tricyclic antidepressant drugs are toxic in small quantities, particularly to the heart, so these children may need treatment in a paediatric intensive care unit.

Head Injury

Shirley was a healthy 7-year-old girl who had had no previous serious illnesses. She lived with her parents and four brothers and two sisters in a three-bedroomed council maisonette which was part of a new property development. The council estate was only partly completed and a planned play area for children was not yet open. Consequently the local children were obliged to play on waste areas and in the street. On a summer evening Shirley was playing ball with an older brother and two friends on a flat piece of waste land close to a busy street. They had been told frequently not to play there, but were unsupervised—Shirley's mother had gone to work and her father was watching television. Inevitably the ball was kicked onto the street. Shirley, in her excitement, went into the street behind a parked car in order to retrieve it. She was struck a glancing blow on the shoulder and head by a van. The driver of the van was travelling at only about 20 miles per hour but nevertheless was not able to stop in time.

Shirley was lying in the street unconscious when the ambulance arrived a few minutes later. The ambulancemen noted that she was breathing without evidence of obstruction of her airway and had easily palpable peripheral pulses.

When examined in the accident and emergency department she was semiconscious, making unco-ordinated movements of the limbs when disturbed. A scalp laceration was present over the left temporal area, but there were no signs of injury to other areas. A skull x-ray showed a fracture in the occipital bone and she was admitted to the children's intensive care unit.

Her general condition settled over the next 12 hours, although her conscious level remained unchanged. However, during the next night there was a deterioration in level of consciousness, associated with bradycardia and hypertension. There was no papilloedema but it was assumed that she had raised intracranial pressure. She was therefore electively ventilated to reduce arterial CO_2, which reduces cerebral blood flow, and given a bolus of intravenous mannitol. An emergency CT brain scan showed diffuse cerebral oedema with no sign of a major intracerebral bleed, so this management was continued for several days.

At the time of discharge from hospital two months later Shirley was well and there were no abnormal neurological signs.

Comment

Fortunately most head injuries to children are mild, but where there has been a period of unconsciousness, hospital admission for 24 hours is a wise precaution. Skull x-rays are not necessary for all head injuries seen in accident and emergency departments, but a

Table 10.5

Signs of raised intracranial pressure following injury (caused by cerebral oedema or intracranial bleeding)

Decreasing level of consciousness
Development of focal neurological signs (particularly unequal pupils)
Rising blood pressure
Falling heart rate

Table 10.6

Late effects of head injury

Mental handicap
Motor handicap (cerebral palsy)
Epilepsy
Personality changes
Depression
Recurrent headaches

skull fracture or scalp injury will suggest the possibility of underlying brain injury. Acceleration–deceleration forces act on the brain as a whole so there is a widespread diffuse injury, and this type of injury from a fall or blunt trauma is the most common in children. Where there is a severe head injury, other injuries may occur and there may be secondary brain damage from hypovolaemic shock or oxygen deprivation.

Most head injuries get better by themselves but careful nursing observation is mandatory to detect clinical deterioration or signs of raised intracranial pressure (Table 10.5). Neurosurgical centres now tend to monitor the pressure directly from the extradural or subarachnoid space (normal < 15 mm Hg) in major brain trauma. Hyperventilation, intravenous mannitol, steroids and hypothermia effectively reduce intracranial pressure, and will prevent tentorial herniation (coning).

CT scanning which now has a high resolution has revolutionized management, as the clinical signs of a haematoma, whatever its site, are largely similar (Fig. 10.10). They result from the combination of focal

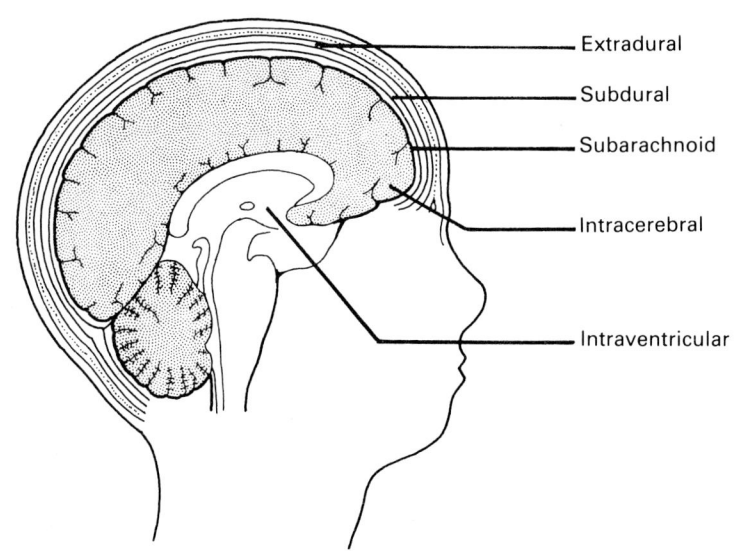

Fig. 10.10
Sites of cerebral bleeding following trauma

compression of the cerebral hemisphere, raised intracranial pressure and coning. When the clinical deterioration is very rapid, burr holes may be indicated if there is no time for a scan.

Clearly there is little that can be done about large cerebral lacerations or diffuse injury. Late effects of head injury (Table 10.6) may be difficult to treat, and the family will be especially distressed if there are personality changes. In head injuries in young children where the explanation is considered inadequate, the possibility of non-accidental injury must always be considered.

11 Behavioural problems

Temper Tantrums

John, an only child who was 2½ years old, caused his parents considerable anxiety because of his behavioural problems and temper tantrums. His temper became apparent at 7 months when he would scream if put down to sleep. More recently he would scream and refuse to eat at meal times unless he could sit on his mother's lap. Even then it usually took about an hour to feed him. John's behaviour generally deteriorated towards the end of the day when tired. Bedtimes were usually very fraught as John would rarely settle and go to sleep by himself but would scream if his mother left him alone. John's father thought he should be left to cry rather than being placated and consoled, but in practice his wife found this impossible to carry out.

A further aspect of John's behaviour which his mother found most upsetting was during her weekly trips to the local supermarket. John always wanted to have several types of sweets at the check-out counter and if he did not get these he would stamp his feet, scream and lie on the floor kicking his legs. This theatrical performance usually attracted an audience and John's mother would leave the shop in tears after criticism from other customers.

Comment

This type of behaviour is very common in this age group—'the terrible twos'. All children have temper tantrums at one time or another during their formative years. Between the ages of 2 and 4 years some degree of negativism, such as refusal to sleep, eat or conform, is a normal part of development of the child's individual personality. These lead to the common behavioural problems of the toddler (Table 11.1) who wants to stand up for himself and resist domination. Sometimes the parents have unreal expectations for the behaviour of their 2 year old and may have rigid and obsessional traits, with little insight into their problems. Generally, attempts at bribery, bullying or coaxing will have failed.

Advice may be sought from a number of places (Fig. 11.1). Management initially consists of taking a full medical and social history in a relaxed environment. The realization that this problem is very common, and having someone to listen to all the details, will go some way to relieving the family tension and anxiety. Clearly a plan of action such as behaviour modification needs to be worked out with both parents so that both are working together in the same direction.

Table 11.1
Common behavioural problems in toddlers

Temper tantrums
Sleep refusal
Food refusal
Breath-holding attacks
Head banging
Toilet refusal

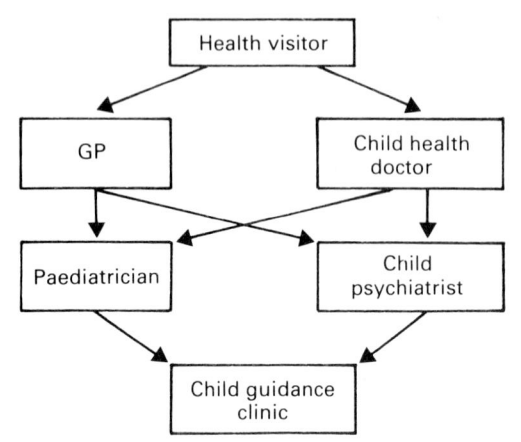

Fig. 11.1
Sources of treatment for behavioural problems

The mealtimes were initially discussed. It was suggested that John be given his food, which he could refuse if he wanted. All attempts to force or coerce food into him were stopped—these are generally doomed to failure, giving the child an immediate upper hand! In this way the attention-seeking gain is removed and the behaviour tends to improve. Temper tantrums with a child lying on the floor screaming, biting and kicking are similarly best ignored (this is easier in theory than in practice!). It is essential that the goal for the objectionable behaviour is never achieved, as this reinforces the behaviour pattern.

John remained a somewhat pampered only child, who did dominate and bully other children. His attention-seeking, self-centred behaviour persisted but this bombastic facade readily crumbled under stress, showing a basic lack of maturity. Can you think of any adults with this type of behaviour pattern?

Overactive Child

Raina, a 3-year-old Indian child, was referred to a paediatric outpatient clinic because of overactive behaviour which her mother found difficult to tolerate. She commented that Raina was a busy child, who was always into everything, and that she would not sit and play by herself for more than a few minutes. Raina had no brothers or sisters and was looked after by a child minder during the day, as her mother worked in the accounts section of the family business. Towards the end of the interview it became clear that the pregnancy had been unplanned and her mother had difficulty adjusting her busy life after Raina's birth.

The child's behaviour was observed carefully from the time she entered the room. Although a busy child moving from one new toy to another, her attention span seemed reasonable. With persistence it was possible to get co-operation from the child to copy building towers and bridges with bricks, and to draw some faces. In fact her developmental and neurological assessment revealed no deficit and most milestones were ahead of those expected, rather than behind.

Her mother was keen for some sedative to be prescribed to improve her uncontrollable behaviour pattern. This was resisted and it was suggested to her mother that more time should be spent with Raina, particularly concentrating on playing and reading. It was felt that one of the factors involved in the child's behaviour was too little stimulation at home, and boredom. This advice was not too well received, but follow-up two months later did show some improvement.

Comment

Some children are relentlessly overactive so that they have ceaseless tireless movements, sleep very little and are readily distracted, with a brief attention span even under optimal conditions. These extrovert characters are impulsive and may expose themselves to

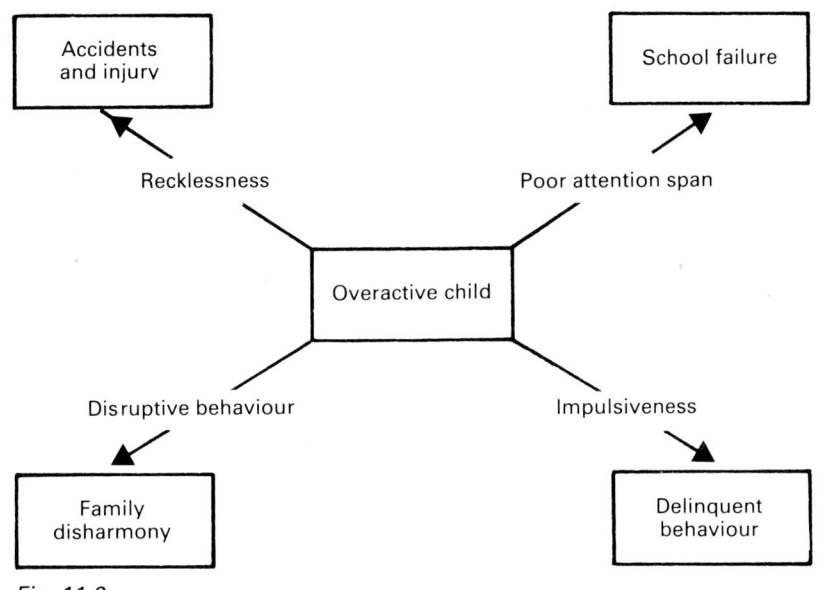

```
        Accidents                          School failure
        and injury
            ↑                                    ↑
     Recklessness                    Poor attention span
                    ┌──────────────┐
                    │Overactive child│
                    └──────────────┘
     Disruptive behaviour            Impulsiveness
            ↓                                    ↓
         Family                          Delinquent
       disharmony                         behaviour
```

Fig. 11.2
Consequences of overactive behaviour

dangers such as road traffic or drowning. Other consequences of such behaviour are shown in Fig. 11.2. Fortunately, such children (who are frequently mentally handicapped) are rare, but less severe forms of overactive behaviour are commonly seen, resulting in referral for advice from schools, doctors, social workers or child guidance clinics. Phenobarbitone is a well known cause of hyperactivity in young children.

There are a number of possible approaches to treatment (Table 11.2). In Raina's case it was clear that maternal rejection and boredom were associated factors, so it was felt more appropriate to direct therapy at the mother, rather than the child. Often behaviour therapy is at least as effective as drug treatment and such techniques can easily be taught to nursery nurses or teachers. These essentially consist of prompt, consistent and acceptable rewards for specified patterns of behaviour. The prognosis is good when the child's IQ is normal and the overactivity is confined to one area of behaviour. With the more severe intractable forms personality development may be affected, so school failure and impulsive behaviour as an adult may ensue.

Table 11.2
Treatment of overactivity in young children

Behaviour modification techniques
Relief of boredom (play group, day nursery, nursery school)
Stopping phenobarbitone
Occasional resort to specific drug therapy (e.g. methylphenidate), especially in mentally handicapped children

Teenage Suicide

Mandy, aged 14, was the least successful of her classmates at school. She missed much school by playing truant and would wander off by herself during school hours. Her father, who was an unemployed welder, was not interested in whether Mandy attended school or not, and he had thrown the education welfare officer out of his house on two occasions. Mandy's mother was a quiet withdrawn woman, who had difficulty coping at home and had a schizoid personality. She seemed to live in a world of her own most of the time and certainly was not interested in Mandy's school attendance or future prospects. She gave little support to her daughter and Mandy frequently had to take over the mothering role by looking after her younger brothers and sisters for days at a time.

Mandy unexpectedly took an overdose during the summer just before arriving at school. She became unconscious during the first lesson of the day and was taken into hospital, where it was subsequently found that she had taken 20 diazepam (Valium) tablets belonging to her mother.

Comment

Suicide is a self-inflicted act resulting in death. Fortunately, it is rare in teenagers, with an incidence of less than 1 in 100 000 cases per year in 10–14 year olds, rising to 5 per 100 000 in 15–19 year olds. Its analogue, parasuicide, where an individual ingests an excessive but not potentially fatal overdose, has an incidence of 500 per 100 000 in 15 year olds, an incidence which has increased tenfold in the last 20 years.

Although these two groups can overlap to some extent, the suicide group shows signs of depression, and are often solitary, intelligent youngsters, culturally distant from their less well educated parents who may be mentally disturbed. The parasuicide group tend to be more aggressive, impetuous children who are immature and sensitive to criticism. Both suicide and parasuicide may be precipitated by stressful life-events such as bereavement, desertion, moving house, unemployment or loss of health. Parasuicide seems to represent impulsive attention-seeking behaviour, particularly in response to an emotional crisis, and is most commonly undertaken with minor tranquillizers—as in adults.

Management plans need to be carefully formulated according to the cause of the attempted suicide. Withdrawn, unhappy children need expert psychiatric assessment and will often need some form of continuing therapy. Emotional parasuicide rarely has a psychiatric basis and the crisis which precipitated it will often resolve spontaneously. Social worker enquiry into the family dynamics is more appropriate in these cases than psychiatric treatment.

Anorexia Nervosa

Jackie, a 12 year old, was admitted to hospital with progressive weight loss over a four-month period, during which time she had lost about 30 per cent of her body weight. Her father, who was a solicitor, had recently found relations between himself and his daughter very strained because of perpetual confrontations during mealtimes. Jackie ate little food and was very fussy in her selection of items, tending to choose fruit and nuts. Her two older brothers, aged 16 and 19 years, who were both rather boisterous teenagers, did not appreciate their meals being disturbed and tended to avoid their younger sister whenever possible. Jackie's mother, an ex-model and lingerie designer, was herself slim and on a strict diet.

Initially there were several visits to the GP who knew the family well. He had carried out a few simple investigations to exclude the possibility of diabetes or thyrotoxicosis and made a clinical diagnosis of anorexia nervosa (Table 11.3). In view of the persistent weight loss he arranged hospital admission with the local paediatrician. Because of Jackie's gross

Table 11.3

Clinical features of anorexia nervosa

Weight loss (more than 25% of expected body weight)
Amenorrhoea
Vomiting
Constipation with laxative abuse
Manipulative behaviour
Secretiveness and hostility
Lack of appreciation of own thinness (distorted body image)

Table 11.4

Example of a treatment plan for an anorexic patient

30 kg	Admission weight
32 kg	Allowed books
34 kg	Allowed portable television
36 kg	Allowed out of bed
38 kg	Parents allowed to visit
40 kg	Sweets allowed
42 kg	Friends allowed to visit
44 kg	Allowed home

emaciation and her manipulative behaviour, a plan of management was drawn up following a discussion with the parents. She was given a cubicle on the ward where she had to stay during her initial hospitalization. No visitors or relatives were allowed to visit for several weeks and all privileges were withdrawn. A 3000 kcal diet was prescribed, avoiding curried foods which she had never eaten. A chart was placed on the wall with target weights for return of privileges (Table 11.4).

Jackie initially appeared to understand the treatment plans and said she would co-operate, but a few nasogastric tube feeds were required to achieve the initial weight gain. The nursing staff caught Jackie vomiting into her sink one night, so this had to be blocked off and more careful observation carried out. After 7 weeks' progressive weight gain her parents were allowed to visit for short periods. The help and advice of a child psychiatrist was sought and he undertook both family therapy and psychotherapy with Jackie. It became apparent after several sessions that there were marriage problems and that the parents were staying together for the sake of the children. The psychiatrist felt that part of the explanation for Jackie's illness was 'her subconscious desire to weld her parents together by creating special demands that needed their attention'.

Comment

The disease is one of western civilization and the frequency increases as one ascends the social scale. It affects females 20 times more often than males. Often because of deceit, much fruitless time can be spent on the investigation of metabolic and endocrine disorders before a psychogenic basis to the illness is suspected. Many girls go through a phase of transient anorexia at times of emotional turmoil when dieting gets out of hand. Distortion of body image and the wish to remain a child rather than achieving womanhood are features of the younger anorexic.

A long duration and the association of vomiting, binge eating or purging are some of the many factors that indicate a less favourable prognosis. In the treatment, manipulation by playing off one member of staff against another should be avoided. In general, discussion about food and weight are initially avoided, except to give target weights. The treatment plan outlined in this case is just one of many alternative methods of management.

12 Surgery

Congenital Dislocation of the Hip

Joanne was born at term by a breech delivery which was uneventful. She had a birth weight of 3.05 kg. During the routine neonatal examination the houseman thought the left hip was abnormal. She performed Barlow's test (Fig. 12.1), during which the thighs were

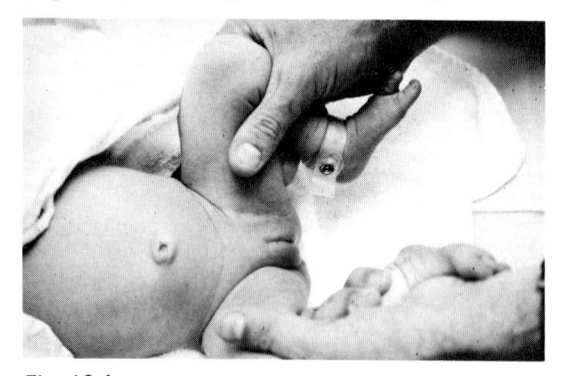

Fig. 12.1
Barlow's test

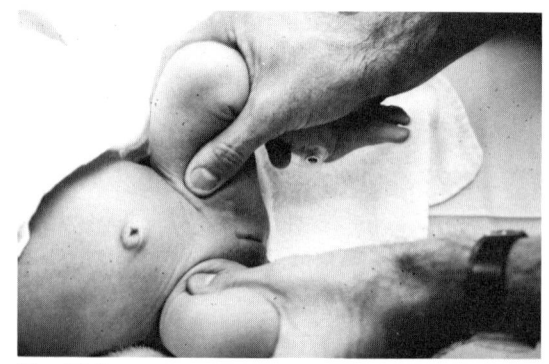

Fig. 12.2
Barlow's test, second part

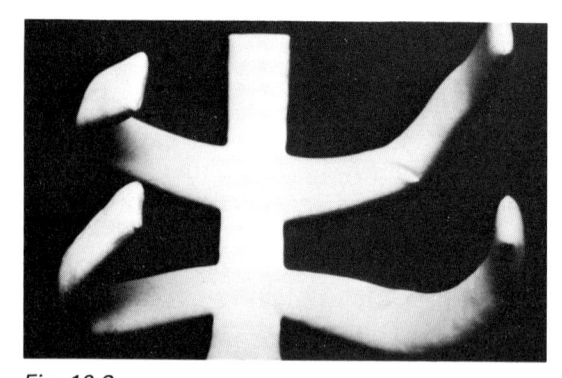

Fig. 12.3
Von Rosen splint

abducted while medial pressure was exerted by the middle fingers on the lateral side of the infant's thigh. The hip was felt to move anteriorly *with a clunk*—i.e. the type of sensation and movement associated with putting a car into gear. The second part of the test (Fig. 12.2) involved adduction with lateral pressure exerted by the thumbs—this produced a posterior movement of the femur *with a clunk*. Joanne therefore had an unstable hip, where the femoral head lay posterior to the acetabulum at rest. The hip could be reduced into the acetabulum and redislocated by pressure on the femur from behind and in front.

These physical signs were confirmed by another experienced examiner and Joanne was referred to an orthopaedic consultant for advice on further management. He treated the child with a Von Rosen splint (Fig. 12.3), which was used for three months to hold the leg in abduction and external rotation. At the end of this time the hips appeared clinically stable and could easily be fully abducted. There was no evidence of rotation of the pelvis or shortening of the leg, and an x-ray of the pelvis showed normal acetabula with the femoral heads in the correct location.

Comment

Congenital dislocation of the hips (CDH) is common. Prior to the introduction of neonatal screening programmes all cases presented late, usually during the first few years of life with symptoms such as limp, leg shortening, difficulty in crawling or external rotation of the foot. The physical signs in cases presenting late are limited abduction, shortening of the leg, waddling gait or telescoping of the leg, so parents' concerns should be taken seriously if the diagnosis is not to be delayed even further. Neonatal screening, originally introduced by Ortolani in Italy in 1948, aims to diagnose potential problems, which are dealt with by splinting for a few months. The success of this programme varies depending on the skill of the examiners, and the incidence of late CDH ranges from 0.1 to 0.6 per 1000.

The newborn examination detects 12 per 1000 hips that are unstable. Clearly the majority of these resolve spontaneously, but it is impossible to predict which of these will develop a complete dislocated hip, even though specific risk factors are known (Table 12.1). The evidence that splinting prevents the dislocatable hip becoming completely and permanently dislocated is very strong. All these cases identified on screening will be followed up and have a pelvic x-ray at about 4 months, when the femoral heads are sufficiently ossified to assess their congruity.

Treatment of the occasional child where

Table 12.1
Risk factors for congenital dislocation of the hips

Positive family history
Girls
Extended breech presentation at birth
Neurological abnormalities (e.g. spina bifida, cerebral palsy)

splinting fails, or of the more common late presentation, involves traction and splintage, usually followed by operative intervention to reduce the dislocation or reconstruct the acetabulum. The morbidity in such children is high; multiple operations may be needed and the child left with a limp or unable to participate in sport. Careful neonatal screening should reduce these late cases to a minimum, but even the most careful examination cannot detect every case.

Cleft Palate and Cleft Lip

Philip was a term baby born with the aid of a pair of forceps, who was noted to have a cleft lip and palate at birth (Fig. 12.4). The cleft was complete, extending from the right nostril to the back of the palate. The paediatric registrar who was on call met the parents, discussed the nature of the defect and checked the baby over for other congenital malformations. He was able to reassure the parents that the defect appeared an isolated one.

The sister from the plastic surgical ward came to see the parents and she demonstrated some practical techniques of feeding the baby and showed the parents photographs of other children before and after repair operations. Because of the relatively large size of the defect, a dental plate was fitted by the oral surgeon so that feeding could be accomplished without regurgitation of milk into the nose (Fig. 12.5). Elastic strapping was also

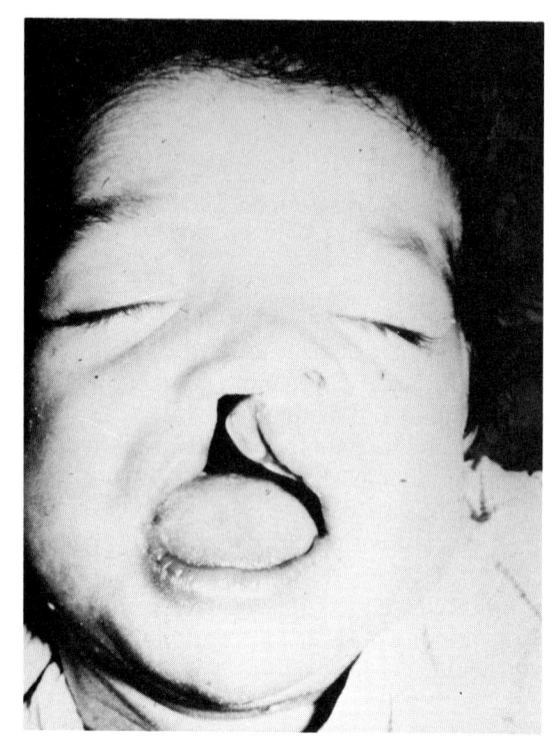

Fig. 12.4
Cleft lip and palate

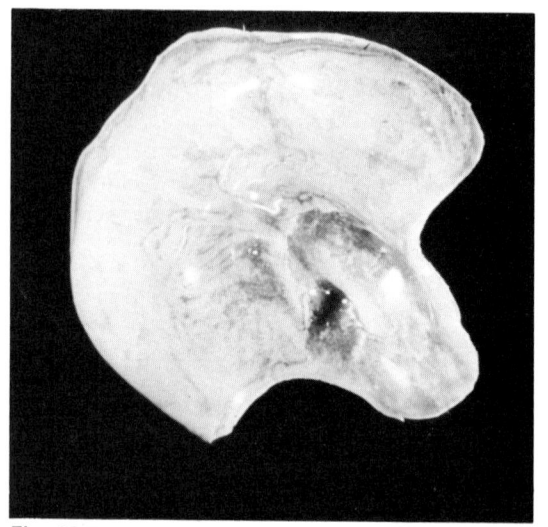

Fig. 12.5
Dental plate

applied across the defect in the lip to encourage the maxillary processes to grow together so that the defect would be reduced in size by the time of surgery (Fig. 12.6).

A plastic surgeon closed the cleft lip at 3 months and repaired the palate at 15 months. Although the repair was cosmetically satisfactory, Philip's speech was difficult to under-

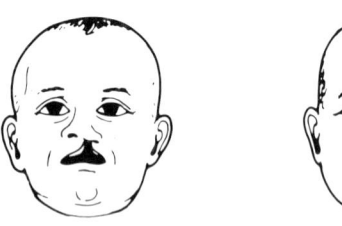

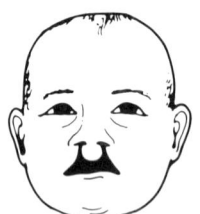

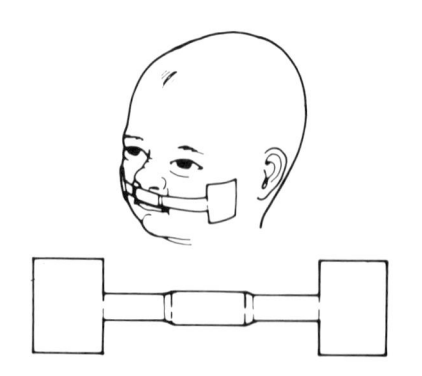

Fig. 12.6
Elastic strapping to face (*From Milner AD & Hull D (1984)* Hospital Paediatrics. *Churchill Livingstone, Edinburgh, by courtesy of the publishers*)

stand because of poor articulation. Since the speech therapist felt she was getting nowhere, further assessment was carried out. An ENT surgeon found a moderate conductive hearing loss (40 dB) which was due to glue ears, and it was felt that his speech sounds were abnormal because of this as well as an air leak from the mouth into the nose. Middle ear drainage with grommets and a secondary operation on the muscles of the soft palate helped somewhat to improve his speech.

Comment

Clefts of the lip and palate arise because of failure of fusion of the median nasal process with the lateral nasal or maxillary processes at 8 weeks' gestation. Cleft palate and/or lip have an incidence of 1 in 500 births. Fortunately, isolated cleft lips (previously called hare lips) are more common than cleft palates, and even bilateral cleft lips can usually be repaired with good cosmetic results. In the management of these children a team approach is helpful; initially most concerns will inevitably focus around feeding and whether a satisfactory cosmetic repair is possible.

It is believed that correct treatment within the first three months of life is crucial to the future success of the child, and so co-operation should be enlisted from parents if the full potentials of treatment are to be achieved. A health visitor who can visit the family at home will prove invaluable if she has had specific training in this area. It is wise to give the parents some advice on the risk of a similar event occurring in future children, and these risks are greater if more than one child is affected.

Irritable Hip

Samantha, a 6 year old, was seen in the accident and emergency department with a left-sided limp and pains in her leg, which had come on over a period of several days. She had otherwise been well in herself and had been at school until the previous day. On direct questioning there was no history of trauma or previous hip problems, and at examination there were limited hip movements in all directions, especially abduction and internal rotation. There was no evidence of other joint involvement, pyrexia or systemic involvement. Samantha was not keen to bear weight on her left leg, but could just walk unaided, albeit wih a limp.

The following investigations were undertaken—full blood count with differential, throat swab and hip x-rays. Apart from a neutrophilia these were normal, and there were no x-ray features to suggest Perthes' disease. Samantha was discharged home with a diagnosis of transient synovitis of the hip, and asked to take simple analgesics and rest her leg.

Comment

Children with pains in the leg or limp are frequently seen in accident and emergency departments or by general practitioners. Accurate diagnosis is essential (Fig. 12.7), as the types of treatment necessary will vary

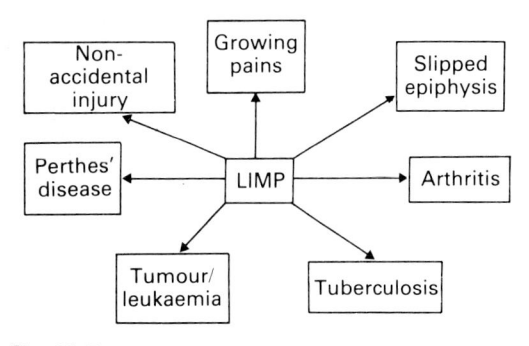

Fig. 12.7

Differential diagnosis in child with a limp

widely. Transient synovitis of the hip is seen in children from 18 months to 12 years and often follows a respiratory infection. Diagnosis is based on the history, refusal to weight bear and pain, together with limitation of abduction and internal rotation of the hip joint. It is impossible to distinguish clinically between transient synovitis and Perthes' disease, making x-rays essential. Related factors to transient synovitis are infection, trauma and obesity, and it should be remembered that the condition is often recurrent.

Treatment is symptomatic with simple analgesia with paracetamol or aspirin and rest. For more severe cases, bed rest with a few days' limb traction may be necessary to relieve pain. The condition is self-limiting after a week or so, and the prognosis is good—as long as the initial diagnosis was correct.

Hypospadias

Garry had a routine neonatal examination during his first day of life and the paediatric houseman noticed that his urethral meatus opened onto the undersurface of the shaft of the penis. In association with this defect, known as hypospadias, he noticed that the foreskin was hooded and that there was a downward curvature of the penis (chordee). During the rest of the examination he noted that both testes were palpable in the scrotum and that the kidneys did not appear enlarged. Observation of the stream of urine revealed no obstruction to flow at the urethral meatus and the rest of the examination was normal.

Naturally the mother was upset at these findings; she had actually noticed the abnormality but was too scared to tell anyone. The houseman and paediatric surgeon spent a long time with the mother, explaining that surgical repair would be necessary and that it would require two or more operative procedures. It was mentioned that the unsightly foreskin should not be circumcised as it would probably be needed for the final definitive repair.

Comment

Hypospadias is a common abnormality occurring in 1 in 300 males. The site of the urethral meatus enables the defect to be classified into mild, moderate or severe (Fig. 12.8) and

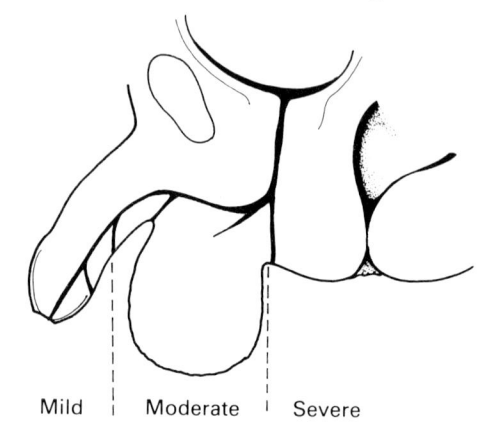

Fig. 12.8
Types of hypospadias

Garry's defect was a moderate hypospadias. With increasing severity of the defect the incidence of other congenital malformations of the urogenital tract increases. Fortunately, about 80 per cent of hypospadias open onto the glans and are therefore a mild defect not requiring treatment, as urine stream, sexual function and potency will not be significantly impaired.

In the more severe defects the distal urethra is represented by a fibrous cord, which leads to the flexion deformity—chordee—which may become more conspicuous during erection. With this type of defect the boy will be incapable of passing urine standing up and this is not socially or psychologically acceptable. Thus, during surgical repair two objects should be achieved. First, the chordee must be straightened and secondly the urethra reconstructed to reach the glans. A number of operations have been devised for both procedures but the Denis Browne repair is commonly used for the latter.

When dealing with the severe type of defect that opens onto the perineum, an intersex state should be excluded by palpation of the testes. If there is doubt about the presence of these, then full endocrinological work-up is indicated, including chromosome analysis for genetic sexing, and serum 17-hydroxy-progesterone measurement to exclude congenital adrenal hyperplasia. Generally a more guarded prognosis is given with these types of defects because the results of surgery are not so good.

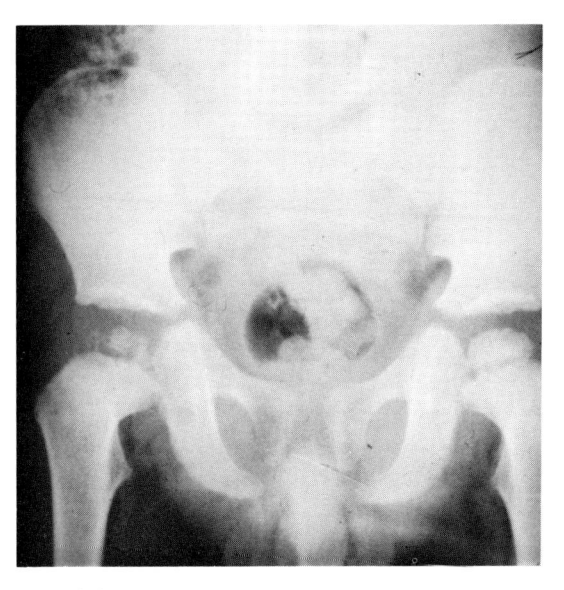

Fig. 12.9
Bilateral Perthes' disease

Perthes' Disease

David, a 5 year old described by his parents as an active busy child, was seen by his doctor because of pains in his right knee. Examination of the knee revealed no abnormality and the parents were reassured that all was well. A month later the parents returned with their son, who had an occasional limp after riding his bicycle. Again the parents were reassured, but they demanded to see an orthopaedic surgeon.

By the time David was seen he had a pronounced limp and pain in his right upper leg. Examination of the hip joint revealed limited abduction and internal rotation of his right leg. The quadriceps muscle above the knee was visibly wasted. A pelvic x-ray was taken (Fig. 12.9) which showed erosion and destruction of the head of the right femoral epiphysis with irregularity of the left epiphysis. These clinical and x-ray signs were felt to be typical of Perthes' disease, which usually involves one hip rather than both simultaneously. The child was put on bed rest until a varus rotation femoral oesteotomy was carried out on the right hip. Physiotherapy and mobilization followed once the plaster of Paris was removed eight weeks later. Regular follow-up was instituted, but an ischial weight-bearing caliper was avoided because of active disease in the opposite joint.

Comment

Perthes' disease is caused by an ischaemic necrosis of the femoral head affecting the epiphysis. The process continues for one or two years, leading to flattening and shrinking of the ossification centre and widening of the femoral neck. Repair takes place over the subsequent two or three years, although permanent damage may produce osteoarthritis.

Typically the disease presents with limp or pain in the leg/knee in children between 7 and 10 years (Fig. 12.10). Treatment is still controversial and difficult to assess because

Onset 3-10 yrs

Male/Female ratio 4:1

10% of cases bilateral

Present as limp ± pain (may be referred to knee)

Hip held flexed and adducted

Muscle wasting often present

Fig. 12.10
Features of Perthes' disease

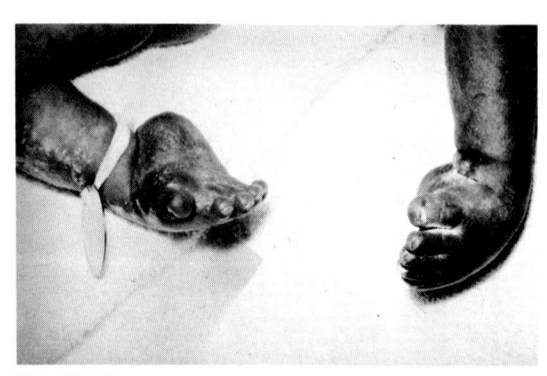

Fig. 12.11
Talipes equinovarus

surgical procedures to assist revascularization have been unsuccessful. Rotation osteotomies and abduction by plaster seem to produce the best results, with least side effects.

Talipes

Angus, a newborn infant, was found to have abnormal feet at his routine neonatal examination. Both were inturned from the ankle (Fig. 12.11), such that the paediatric houseman was unable to even partially correct this deformity. The infant's toes could not be placed on the front of his shin. Examination of the baby, with particular attention to the back and nervous system excluded any other deficit.

The baby was then referred to an orthopaedic surgeon, who noted that the feet were in fixed plantar flexion (equinus), with inversion of the heel and foot (varus) and adduction of the forefoot. These are the findings of talipes equinovarus (club foot). For the first few days, leg manipulation exercises were given but serial corrective plaster casts were then used in an attempt to correct the deformity. After a few months, operative treatment was undertaken to release soft tissues and tendons on the medial side of the feet. The equinus position of the feet persisted, and at a later operation the Achilles tendons were lengthened. There appeared to be reasonable function without pain as long as special fitted shoes were used, but a total correction had not been achieved.

Comment

The condition has an incidence of 1 in 1000 and is commoner in boys than girls; it is bilateral in 50 per cent of cases. A positional defect with the superficial appearance of talipes is common, but such feet are easily manually

of the long natural history of the disease and the tendency for spontaneous improvement. The aims of treatment have generally been to reduce weight bearing on the hip and to maintain the head in the acetabulum. Bed rest for months or years is currently out of vogue, and correctable and do not require specific treatment. In the older child, talipes may be secondary to a neurological deficit such as that caused by spina bifida, cerebral palsy or polio.

Treatment is difficult but few surgeons have any doubt that the management in the first year is critical to success. The problems of treatment centre around the correction of a deformity which is in three planes and involves several joints simultaneously during a time of rapid growth. In severe cases the talus will be small and underdeveloped.

Tendon transfers from one side of the foot to the other may be necessary to restore balance to the foot. As discussed, lengthening procedures on tendons may also be needed. Treatment that is unsuccessful in early years will leave the grown child with a painful foot that is stiff and deformed, resulting in poor function, so there will be difficulty running, crossing rough terrain or even climbing a ladder. Arthrodesis of ankle or foot joints may become necessary at a late stage. Fortunately, simple treatment measures are often effective during the early months of life. Club foot, which is basically of unknown aetiology, still represents a major challenge to the orthopaedic surgeon.

Wilms' Tumour

John, a 3 year old, was seen in the outpatient clinic as a new patient with a history of weight loss and abdominal pain which had appeared over several weeks. His mother commented that the referring doctor had not examined John's abdomen. John was usually a well child, who had not had any past medical history of note. Abdominal examination revealed gross distension and the presence of superficial veins which were easily visible (Fig. 12.12). A hard mass, which just crossed the midline, was palpable on the left side of the abdomen.

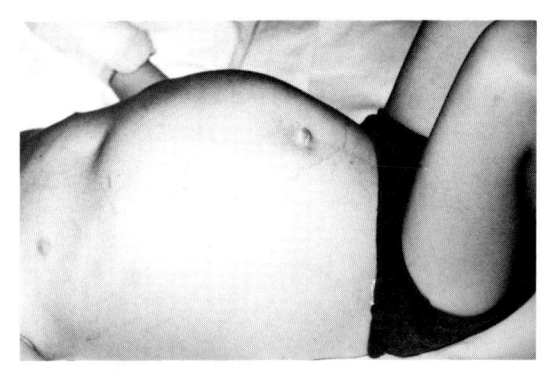

Fig. 12.12
Abdominal mass

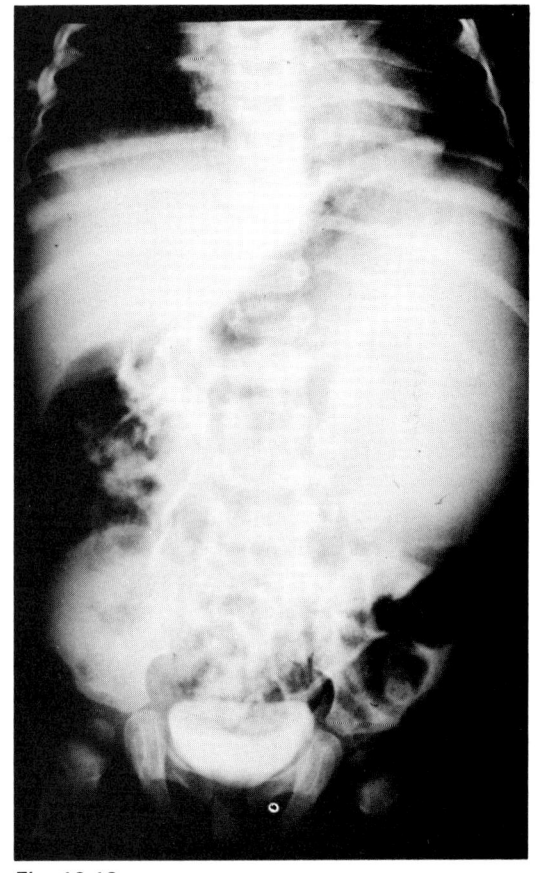

Fig. 12.13
Intravenous urogram showing left-sided renal mass

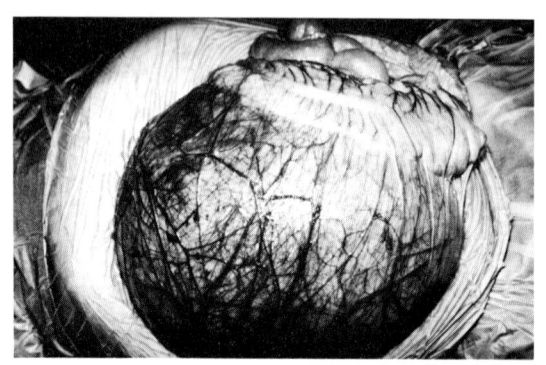

Fig. 12.14
Wilms' tumour found at operation

Table 12.2
Staging of Wilms' tumour

Stage I	Tumour limited to kidney and excised
Stage II	Tumour extends beyond kidney but is excised
Stge III	Residual intra-abdominal tumour after surgery
Stage IV	Metastases in lung, liver, bone or brain
Stage V	Bilateral tumour at diagnosis

Hospital admission was arranged for investigation and treatment. Initially abdominal ultrasound was carried out, and this showed a mass arising from the left kidney. An intravenous urogram confirmed this and showed a large renal mass on the left side which did not excrete any dye (Fig. 12.13). These findings were thought to be typical of a nephroblastoma (Wilms' tumour), rather than a tumour arising from the adrenal gland itself. A number of other investigations, including a chest x-ray looking for lung secondaries, were normal.

Radiotherapy and chemotherapy were commenced in order to diminish tumour volume, facilitate nephrectomy and prevent later surgical spillage of tumour cells. Radiotherapy was given to the left renal bed and the drugs administered were intravenous vincristine and actinomycin. Two weeks later, after another dose of vincristine, a left nephrectomy was undertaken through a large transabdominal incision and the left kidney and tumour were excised (Fig. 12.14). All residual tumour inside the abdomen was removed at surgery and the right kidney was palpated to exclude a bilateral tumour, which is present in 10 per cent of cases. The tumour was designated as stage II (Table 12.2) with favourable histology.

Comment

There are about 70 new cases of this embryonal tumour in the UK each year, making up about 5 per cent of cases of childhood malignancy. Treatment involves a combination of surgery, radiotherapy and chemotherapy given according to a specific protocol. The results of treatment have dramatically improved in recent years so that children with stage I tumours now have a six-year survival of nearly 90 per cent, whereas those with stage IV disease achieve a 40 per cent survival. Such results are obtained from regional units specializing in paediatric oncology, where sufficient multidisciplinary expertise is available to obtain optimal results.

13 Skin disorders

Nappy Rash

Shaun, aged 8 weeks, was the first of identical twins who were both brought for advice about their nappy rash. The rash covered the whole napkin area, which was bright red with satellite areas on the trunk and legs (Fig. 13.1).

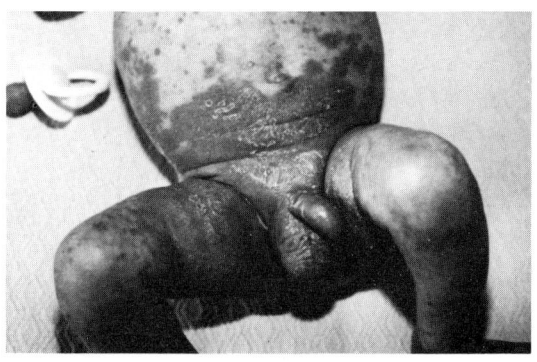

Fig. 13.1
Infantile seborrhoeic eczema

There was also extensive cradle cap (scaling of the scalp), with a scaly rash behind the ears, which was moist and weepy in the cleft between the ears and the scalp. This looked like a secondary bacterial infection (impetiginization) of the rash which was typical of seborrhoeic eczema.

The mother was advised to moisturize the skin by using an aqueous cream in the bath water, and to avoid the use of soap. A local antibiotic cream was applied behind the ears and 1% hydrocortisone cream used for the rest of the skin. The initial response was satisfactory but the rash did not completely disappear from the nappy area so a stronger fluorinated steroid cream—triamcinolone in neomycin and nystatin—was substituted.

Comment

Most babies have a nappy rash at one time or another during the early months of life. Some of these can be prevented by a number of measures (Table 13.1).

Table 13.1
Prevention of nappy rash

Regular changing of wet nappies
Use of nappy liners or disposable nappies
Wash nappy area with warm water when changing nappy
Use of a barrier cream (such as zinc and castor oil)

Infantile seborrhoeic eczema is the commonest rash and the diagnosis is obvious if the whole infant is examined. The lesions on the trunk are characterized by erythema and greasy scales sometimes known as potato chip scales. Treatment involves the use of steroid creams, moisturizing agents and treatment of secondary monilial infection with nystatin cream.

Napkin dermatitis implies some degree of neglect and this may be obvious from the smell and general appearance of the baby before he is undressed. The rash is confined to the nappy area, with sparing of the flexures which are not in contact with wet urine. In grossly neglected infants, ulceration and infection produce an unpleasant rash (Fig. 13.2). Hospital admission and social worker involvement will probably be necessary as well as a combination of steroid, nystatin and antibiotic.

Napkin psoriasis (Fig. 13.3) looks like adult psoriasis with closely demarcated zones. Treatment is similar to the other conditions. About 1 in 6 infants will later develop psoriasis as adults.

Nappy rash can indicate a trivial skin complaint or be the presentation of gross child neglect, so vigilance is needed in the assessment and treatment of this condition.

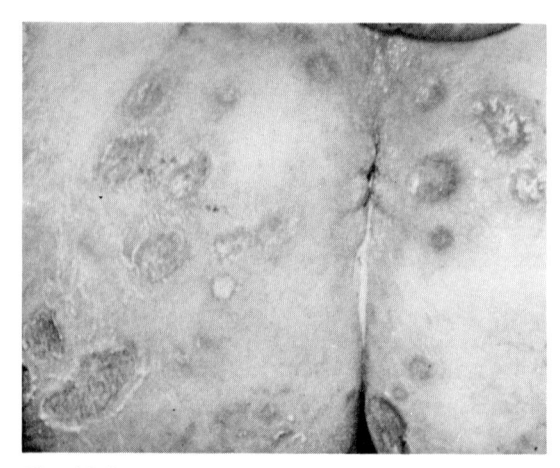

Fig. 13.2
Napkin dermatitis

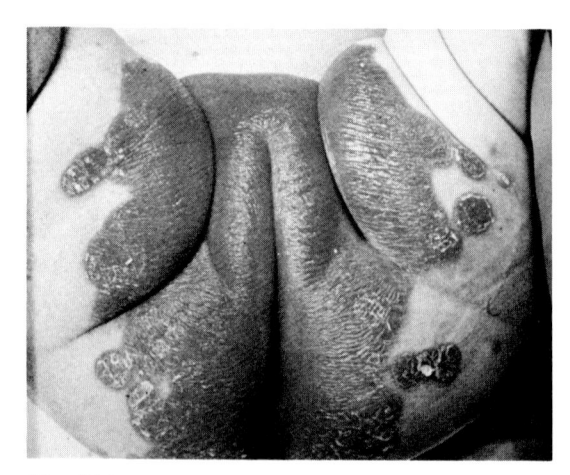

Fig. 13.3
Napkin psoriasis

Atopic Eczema

Nick was seen at 18 months of age with a generalized rash which had been present for many months. His arms, legs and face were mainly involved; these areas were itchy and he tended to scratch and make them bleed. On questioning it became clear that the mother had recurrent attacks of bronchitis, which had recently been labelled as asthma, resulting in a change in her treatment from antibiotics to bronchodilators (which had greatly improved her). There was no other family history of relevance and no obvious factors which provoked Nick's eczema. He was free of any respiratory symptoms.

Examination of the skin showed many dry areas which were excoriated and thickened, with deep fissures over the wrists and hands. Although there was a generalized lymphadenopathy with small shotty nodes, there was no evidence of secondary infection.

The initial management plan suggested avoiding soaps and substituting emulsifying ointment and aqueous cream in the bath water, in an attempt to moisturize the skin. It was suggested that the nails be kept short to reduce skin trauma and bathing frequency kept low to avoid drying the skin. The eczema was treated with 1% hydrocortisone ointment, a weak topical steroid, and a further visit was arranged after a few weeks. By this time there had been some improvement, but the hands and feet were still sore so clobetasone butyrate (Eumovate) ointment was prescribed for these, with specific instructions on the method of administration.

SKIN DISORDERS 135

Outer surfaces | Flexures | Hands and feet

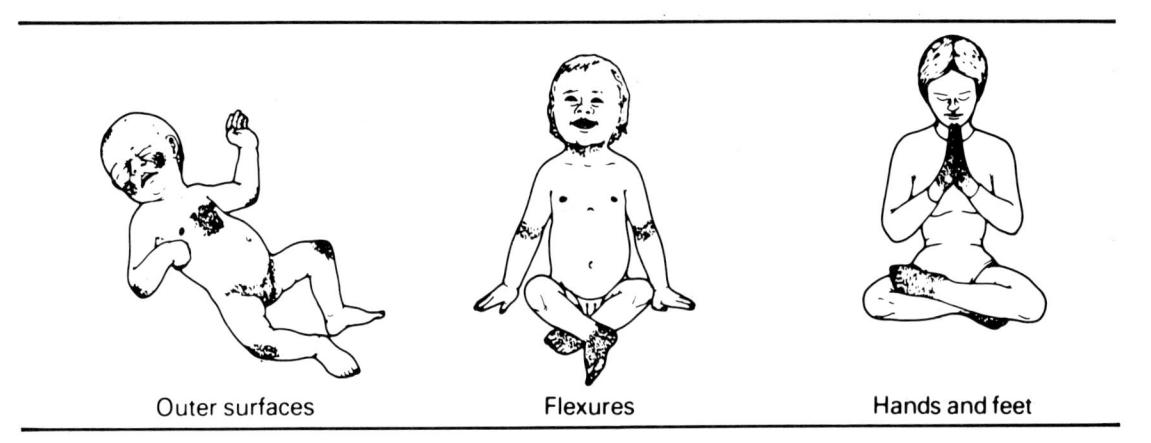

Fig. 13.4
Distribution of infantile eczema (*From Milner AD & Hull D (1984)* Hospital Paediatrics. *Churchill Livingstone, Edinburgh, by courtesy of the publishers*)

Comment

Atopic eczema affects about 5–10 per cent of children. The pathogenesis has not yet been established, although dietary factors and genetic susceptibility have been implicated; for example, there have been suggestions that breast feeding protects the baby against the disease. Atopic eczema is rare in the newborn but has a peak incidence around 5 months of age. It is thought that only 10 per cent of children with infantile eczema will be still affected at adolescence.

Diagnosis is usually easy; the commonly involved sites at different ages are shown in Fig. 13.4. Eczema must be distinguished from seborrhoeic dermatitis, found in the first few months of life, and from psoriasis, where the

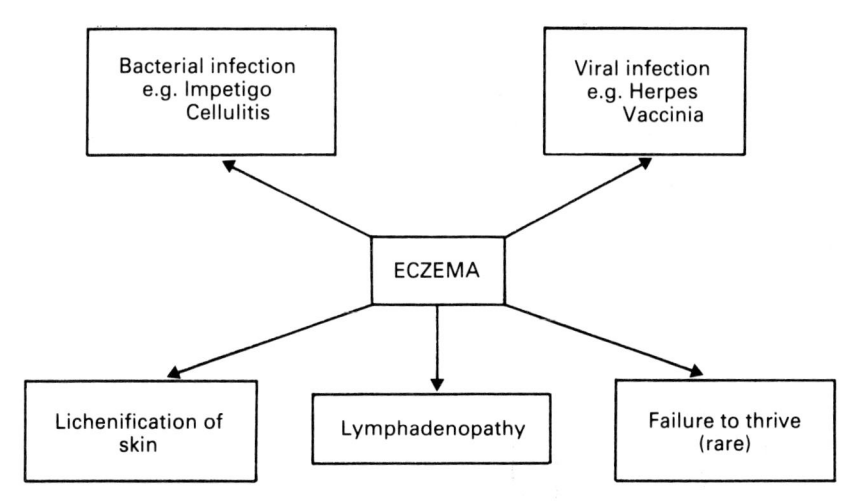

```
         Bacterial infection           Viral infection
         e.g. Impetigo                 e.g. Herpes
         Cellulitis                    Vaccinia
                    \                /
                     \              /
                      →  ECZEMA  ←
                     /     |      \
                    /      |       \
         Lichenification   Lymphadenopathy   Failure to thrive
         of skin                              (rare)
```

Fig. 13.5
Complications of eczema

lesions are much more demarcated. The scalp is frequently involved in psoriasis, whereas eczema predominantly affects the hands and feet, flexures and outer surfaces of the body. There are a number of complications of eczema (Fig. 13.5).

Some aspects of management have already been discussed. The idea is to reduce symptoms and to improve the external appearance by keeping the disease under control. Measures other than topical steroids such as zinc paste and coal-tar bandages can be helpful, but they are avoided in children because such preparations tend to end up on the walls of the home! Topical antihistamines are contraindicated because of skin sensitization but an oral antihistamine at night will reduce itching and help sleep. Since complete cure is not possible until spontaneous remission, second opinions are commonly sought.

Impetigo

Justin was a 4 year old seen because of an extensive rash on his face which failed to respond to hydrocortisone cream. He had never had previous skin problems such as eczema, and there was no family history of atopy. At examination he was a well child who was somewhat dirty. A similar rash was present over his fingers (Fig. 13.6) and both sets of lesions were crusty with moist oozing areas that seemed to be discharging serous fluid. His mother mentioned that another child at the day nursery which Justin attended had 'gone down' with the same rash.

Both children were temporarily removed from the nursery, swabs taken from the lesions and local antibiotic cream of chlortetracycline was applied as well as a course of oral flucloxacillin.

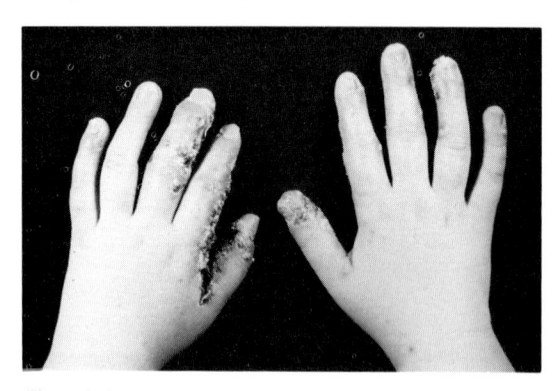

Fig. 13.6
Impetigo of hands

Comment

Impetigo contagiosum is a common superficial skin infection in children caused by *Staphylococcus aureus* or beta-haemolytic streptococcus. The condition is highly contagious and may be the result of a secondary infection of head lice, scabies, cold sores, insect bites or eczema. Most commonly the face, hands, scalp and neck are involved.

The primary lesion is a bulla which fills with pus, ruptures and forms a superficial ulcer. Infected serum oozes from this lesions which the child will spread from one area to another with his fingers. Treatment is with topical antibiotics, after taking a skin swab, and the treatment of any underlying skin condition. Systemic antibiotics are reserved for more severe cases.

Occasionally, impetigo may present as a solitary annular lesion that looks like a cigarette burn—there is a deep ulcerated crater about 0.5 cm across. In this situation it is best to ask for a dermatological opinion before a case conference for suspected non-accidental injury is arranged.

14 Neurological disorders

Infantile Spasms

Anita, a 10 month old, was seen in a children's neurology clinic. Her mother had been concerned about her progress for two or three months, as she seemed to have poor co-ordination, was uninterested in her surroundings and was unable to sit up unsupported. During the two weeks before she was seen she had had a number of bizarre attacks during which her trunk would flex on her hips and her arms extend and abduct. A total of ten of these episodes had been observed.

A detailed history revealed an absence of perinatal problems, family history of fits or mental retardation and that Anita's two elder brothers were fit and well. A developmental examination suggested that Anita was functioning at a level appropriate for a 4 month old, and a neurological examination showed no specific physical signs. On general examination a depigmented patch of skin was seen over the right shin. The neurologist concluded that there was global developmental delay, and that these episodes were convulsions typical of 'salaam attacks' found in a specific type of epilepsy called infantile spasms.

Comment

'Infantile spasms' describe stereotyped fits which are seen in some children aged between 3 and 12 months. Initially there is only a brief loss of postural tone but they evolve rapidly into the classic type already described. A wide variety of structural and metabolic conditions such as asphyxial brain damage or subdural haematomas can underlie the condition. This child was found to have numerous nodules throughout the cerebral cortex on CT scanning, confirming the underlying cause as tuberous sclerosis, and the EEG showed a chaotic pattern (hypsarrhythmia). This dominantly inherited condition was also present in her mother, albeit in much milder form. The diagnosis can often be made from depigmented skin patches, subungual fibromas or the facial rash of adenoma sebaceum. A Wood's ultraviolet light can be used to locate the depigmented patches, found in tuberous sclerosis. None of these features was present in Anita's brothers.

Because the mother is affected, there is a 50:50 chance of another child being affected. However, since the manifestations of the disease are so variable it is impossible to predict whether a future child would be mentally handicapped or merely have a few skin manifestations of the disease. The parents made enquiries about adoption but they were discouraged after they found there was a long waiting list, and in any case they were told they would be given low priority.

Treatment of infantile spasms involves daily ACTH given intramuscularly and also benzodiazepines such as nitrazepam or clonazepam for intractable fits. The prognosis of infantile spasms is not good, especially if there is developmental delay prior to the diagnosis. Prompt diagnosis and the early use of ACTH may prevent subsequent damage in a few cases. Anita was assessed at 4 years and found to be severely mentally handicapped as well as having poorly controlled grand mal epilepsy.

Petit Mal Epilepsy

Carla, a 7 year old girl, was referred to the paediatric outpatient clinic by the school medical officer. During the previous term her school performance had rapidly deteriorated and her teacher was very worried about her progress. She arranged a referral to the doctor, thinking the most likely problem was deafness. When examined at school there were no abnormal neurological signs, her blood pressure was 85/60 mm Hg and her hearing was normal. During the course of the interview the doctor noticed that Carla failed to answer direct questions which he had to repeat before getting an appropriate response.

These findings were confirmed at the hospital. During further assessment Carla was shown how to hyperventilate and during this procedure she suddenly began to stare vacantly at the wall in front of her. It was noticed that her eyelids flickered several times a second, and that she failed to respond to questions during the attack which lasted about ten seconds. An EEG test was performed and this showed a typical 'spike and wave' pattern, typical of petit mal epilepsy, thus confirming the initial clinical impression.

Carla was treated with ethosuximide (30 mg/kg per day), which is used specifically for such attacks, and this enabled their frequency to be reduced to one or two each week. It later became clear that Carla had been having several hundred attacks a week. As expected, school performance improved following control of these fits.

Comment

Petit mal epilepsy is much less common than grand mal, having an incidence of only 12 per 100 000 population. The frequency of attacks is very variable, with a range from the occasional episode to hundreds each day. With a high frequency the child can be reduced to a zombie-like condition, where he is not too sure what is going on in the world around him. Presentation of attacks may be with a behavioural problem or with deteriorating school performance. When a reliable history is not available the induction of attacks by hyperventilation can prove very useful. Alternatively, the classic EEG picture will assist in diagnosis.

The treatment of most types of epilepsy hinges on drug treatment with anticonvulsants, given according to the type of epilepsy. In petit mal epilepsy (classified as a minor type) ethosuximide is given and blood or salivary levels can be used to monitor compliance or to achieve optimal dosage. When petit mal is combined with another form of epilepsy such as grand mal, sodium valproate is a useful alternative drug.

The prognosis for petit mal epilepsy is excellent, and the majority of children will be of normal intelligence and will grow out of their attacks by the time they are teenagers. A more guarded outlook is given when there are different types of fit or atypical EEG appearances.

Grand Mal Epilepsy

Charlene presented to the accident and emergency department at 8 years of age, having had a generalized convulsion at home, lasting between five and ten minutes. Her father said her eyes had become glazed, rolled upwards and she then fell to the ground. Shortly afterwards her arms and legs had begun to shake rhythmically. Charlene also bit her tongue during the attack and was found in a pool of urine. Following the episode she was drowsy and confused and her father had difficulty keeping her awake. When examined an hour after the attack whe was apyrexial and there were no abnormal neurological signs.

Charlene was born at term and had no perinatal problems. There was no relevant past medical history; in particular she had not had any recent head injury or meningitis. Further questioning revealed no family history of epilepsy. No investigations were carried out other than a capillary blood glucose level which was found to be normal.

A follow-up outpatient appointment was made following Charlene's discharge from the accident and emergency department. During the intervening three weeks she had two further fits which were similar to the first. Sodium valproate was commenced as an anticonvulsant and no further fits were seen over the next 18 months. Her school performance continued to be excellent.

Comment

A diagnosis of epilepsy is usually made from the history, as attacks are seldom witnessed by nurses or doctors. Great care in history taking is needed because children can have a wide variety of fits, faints and funny turns (Table 14.1). In the young child, breath-holding attacks are most commonly confused with fits and do not respond to anticonvulsants. Febrile convulsions are also very common in young children and these rarely develop into epilepsy. The majority of childhood epilepsy is idiopathic but secondary causes should be considered, such as cerebral tumours or a degenerative condition. Categorization of epilepsy is helpful in deciding management and prognosis (Table 14.2).

About 4 in 1000 children are considered epileptic by the age of 11 years, and by far the commonest type is grand mal epilepsy (like Charlene). Investigations are rarely helpful in children over a year who have normal developmental progress or intelligence, and in whom focal neurological features are absent. Management includes family support and drug therapy. Serum or salivary drug levels may be helpful in monitoring treatment, which is usually continued for two years from the last fit. Restrictions in everyday activities can be avoided with nocturnal epilepsy, but care should be exercised with the activities listed in Table 14.3 when there is no predictive aura.

Table 14.1
Differential diagnosis of epilepsy

Breath-holding attacks
Reflex anoxic seizures
Simple faints
Febrile convulsions
Behaviour disorders
Recurrent hypoglycaemia
Cardiac arrhythmias
Munchausen's syndrome by proxy

Table 14.2
Clinical types of epileptic attacks

Grand mal (major motor)
Focal (jacksonian)
Temporal lobe (psychomotor)
Infantile spasms
Petit mal

Table 14.3
Restrictions usually imposed on children with epilepsy

No swimming unless accompanied by a responsible adult
No cycling in traffic
No climbing heights

Contrary to popular belief, most children with epilepsy have easily controlled fits and are of normal intelligence. About 85 per cent of children with grand mal epilepsy starting between 1 and 10 years of age will go into remission eventually, so an optimistic outlook can be given to parents.

Mental Handicap

Darren, 2 years old, was seen at his local child health clinic at the request of the health visitor who was concerned about his developmental progress. The mother had not previously attended, so Darren had not had routine immunizations or previous assessment. There had been several changes of housing during the previous year, all around the city centre.

When questioned, the mother remembered Darren first smiled when 12 weeks old, sat up at 8 months and walked by 18 months. She had noted his speech was perhaps slower than expected and it became clear that there were only two comprehensible words spoken ('mumma' and 'no'). He had not learnt to wave bye-bye and did not copy or mimic others. The perinatal history was unremarkable.

When assessed, Darren picked up bricks which he tended to mouth, but could not be coerced into building a tower. Play with miniature toys was similar. He seemed to become bored with a brick after a while and tended to throw it away without any further interest. There was no motor deficit apart from mild generalized hypotonia. Visual acuity was normal, his hearing was normal and a formal assessment by an audiologist was satisfactory. It was felt that the degree of social deprivation was insufficient to account for his developmental delay, although no specific aetiology could be found for his problems.

Periodic follow-up at a multidisciplinary assessment unit was arranged and at 5 years old his IQ was thought to be around 55.

The home was felt to be less stimulating than desirable so a day nursery place was arranged. Nevertheless, his progress remained slow despite the use of a developmental programme carried out by the nursery staff. The educational psychologist prepared a statement of special educational needs with the parents, as it was clear that Darren would be educationally subnormal.

Comment

Developmental assessment in mentally handicapped children during early childhood reveals delay, especially in social and language skills. Intelligence as measured by IQ tests attempts to measure higher intellectual function, which is influenced by genetic and environmental factors. Consistent results are produced from 4 years upwards. A normal distribution of IQ would be expected in the population but there is a slight skew at the lower end because of children with organic brain damage (Fig. 14.1). By definition, mean IQ is 100; and 94 per cent ($\pm 2\,SD$) of the population fall between 70 and 130.

Moderate mental handicap (IQ 50–70) has a prevalence of 3 per cent and is generally due to adverse genetic and psychosocial factors. It is a phenomenon of lower socioeconomic groups (Fig. 14.2). Severe handicap (IQ below 50) is fortunately much less common and is often associated with organic causes (one-third Down's syndrome), with an equal social class distribution.

There are numerous causes of severe handicap which are important for the understanding of prevention. They have been traditionally classified into prenatal, perinatal and postnatal. Preventive measures such as screening for neonatal hypothyroidism and phenylketonuria, and rubella immunizations

Fig. 14.1

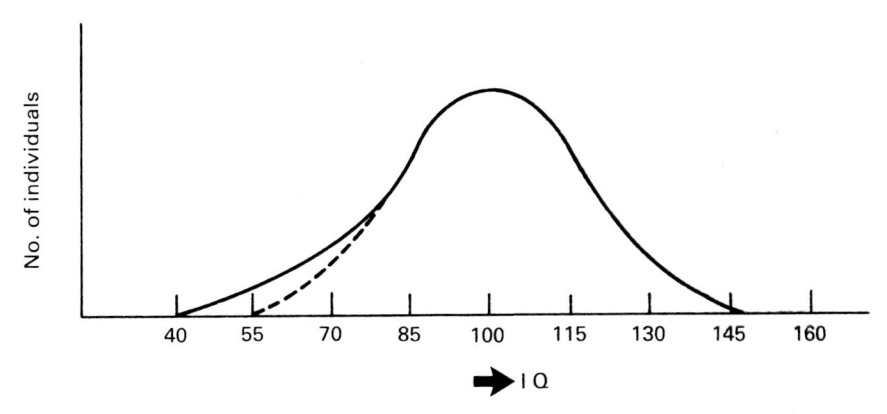

Age distribution of IQ in the population (dotted line normal distribution, solid line actual distribution of IQ)

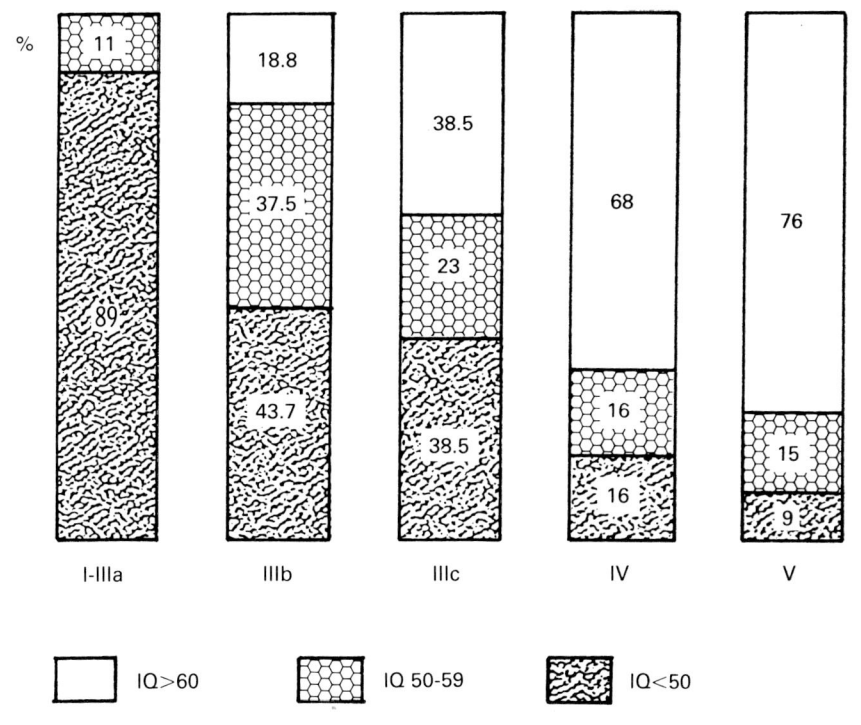

Fig. 14.2

Mental handicap in relation to social class distribution

have been introduced in recent years. Cerebral damage from non-accidental injury may become less frequent if early intervention in such families is possible. Other recent advances include routine amniocentesis for mothers aged over 35 years (which should reduce the incidence of Down's syndrome by a third), and a recognition of X-linked mental handicap with 'fragile sites' on sex chromosomes which enables genetic counselling to be carried out.

The management of severely handicapped children, one-third of whom are institutionalized, has previously been discussed (see Down's syndrome in Chapter 1).

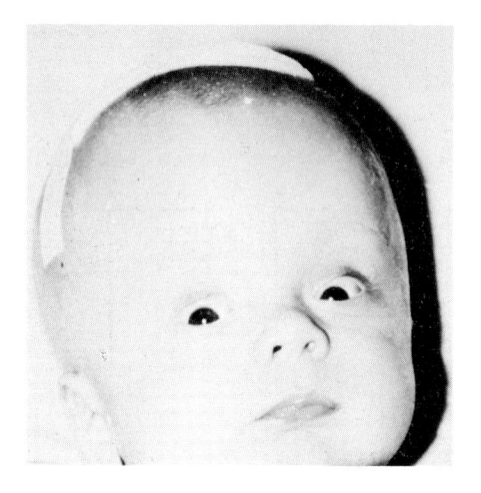

Fig. 14.3
Facies of hydrocephalic child

At examination the head appeared large with a prominent forehead, and the sunset eye sign was present (Fig. 14.3) with the whites of his sclerae visible above the pupils. The anterior fontanelle was large and there was splaying of the sagittal suture. An occipitofrontal head measurement which gives the maximum circumference (Fig. 14.4) was obtained with a tape measure and revealed that the head circumference had gone from the 10th centile at birth to the 90th centile at

OCCIPITO - FRONTAL MEASUREMENT OF HEAD CIRCUMFERENCE

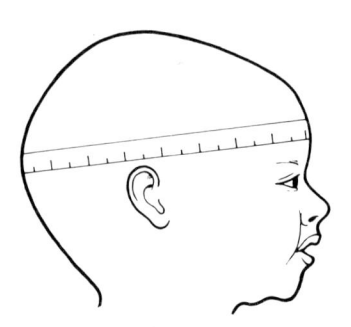

Fig. 14.4
Measurement of head circumference

Hydrocephalus

Paul was brought up to the accident and emergency department by his mother at 4 weeks of age with a history of several days' vomiting and poor feeding. He had been a term baby, weighing 3.16 kg at birth, and had been born following an elective lower segment caesarean section for cephalopelvic disproportion. He had been in good condition at birth and was routinely discharged home on the fourth day. His feeding and weight gain had been satisfactory up until a week prior to being seen in the accident and emergency department.

4 weeks. Paul was admitted to hospital for investigation and treatment.

Initially the infant's head was transilluminated in a dark room while the infant was held by a young nurse and a fibreoptic light shone on the scalp. The investigation, which is very popular with some housemen, distinguishes a large head from subdural haemorrhage, as the latter will not transilluminate. It does not, however, distinguish between hydranencephaly (absent cerebral hemispheres, replaced by fluid) and hydrocephaly (excessive fluid within the ventricles). A CT scan (Fig. 14.5) showed grossly dilated ventricles with normal cerebral cortex surrounding them.

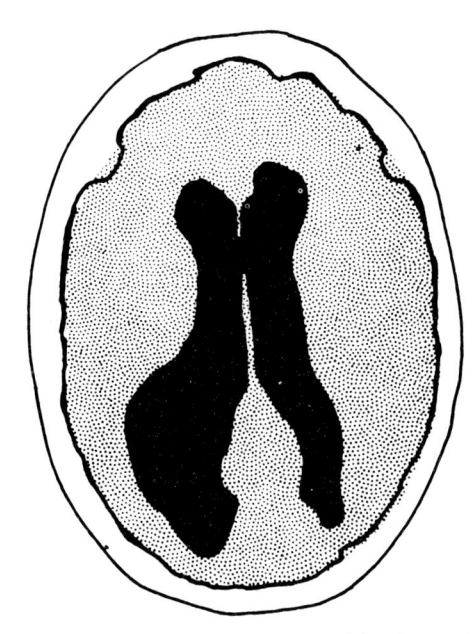

Typical CAT scan appearance of hydrocephalus

Fig. 14.5
Typical CT scan appearance in hydrocephalus

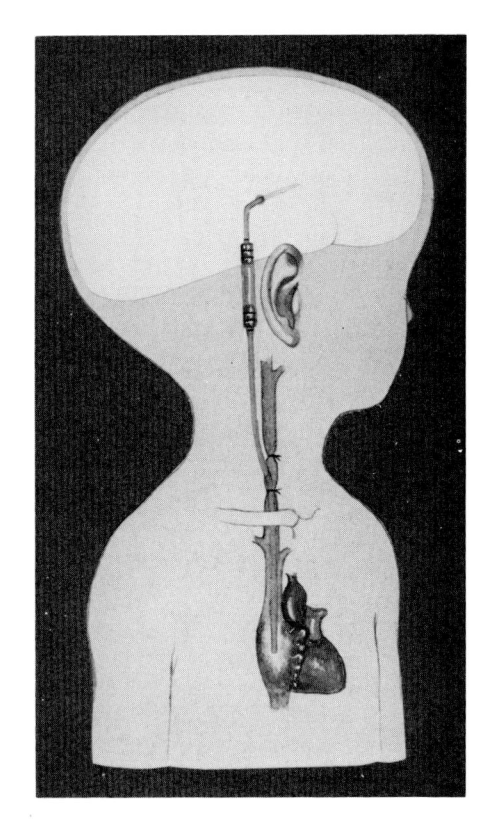

Fig. 14.6
Ventriculoatrial shunt

An emergency shunt operation was carried out by the paediatric surgeon, who performed a ventriculo-peritoneal shunt. This operation was successful and follow-up revealed satisfactory progress. At 2 years developmental progress was normal.

Comment

Hydrocephalus can occur as an isolated defect, as in this case, or may be found in association with other developmental defects such as spina bifida. It can also follow meningitis or an intracranial haemorrhage. For practical purposes CSF production comes from the fronds of the choroid plexus within the cerebral ventricles. The CSF emerges from foramina in the fourth ventricle, and then passes over the surface of the hemispheres prior to absorption by arachnoid villi on the brain surface and along the sagittal sinus. The terms communicating and non-communicating hydrocephalus are of little clinical value, as obstructions may be present at several sites simultaneously.

Early hydrocephalus in children under a year may be detected by serial measurements of head circumference of high-risk babies (i.e. very low birth weight infants) or by the classic features already described. When there is an acute rise in CSF pressure the infant will be lethargic, but irritable when handled and exhibit a high-pitched scream. Papilloedema and bradycardia, commonly seen with raised intracranial pressure in older children and adults, are rarely seen at this age prior to fusion of skull sutures.

system. Complications of shunts are relatively common (Fig. 14.7) and will compromise the eventual quality of life in some children. Fortunately the incidence of spina bifida, an important cause of hydrocephalus, has fallen dramatically since alpha-fetoprotein screening in pregnancy was introduced.

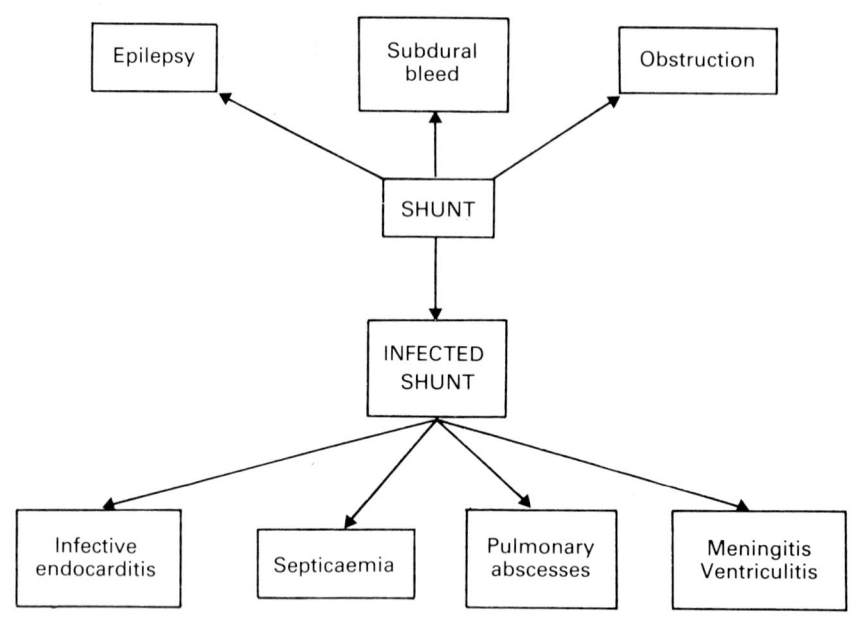

Fig. 14.7
Complications of shunt operations

Real-time ultrasound scanning produces nearly as much information as CT scanning when the anterior fontanelle, which provides an acoustic window, is open, and it is widely used for initial assessment. Modern treatment of hydrocephalus is by diversion of CSF to the peritoneal cavity—a procedure which has fewer complications than a ventriculoatrial shunt (Fig. 14.6). Shunts have valves to prevent reflux of blood or CSF and to control the pressure at which CSF is released. As children grow, shunts tend to pull out of the right atrium or peritoneum, and block. Revision is therefore commonly needed to lengthen the

Duchenne Muscular Dystrophy

Adrian, a 5 year old, was referred by his GP to a paediatrician because of abnormal gait. He had been born at term with a birth weight of 3.40 kg and had not experienced any neonatal problems. His developmental progress had been normal, apart from some delay in his motor milestones (he first walked unaided at 20 months). He had always apparently been rather wobbly on his feet. He was otherwise fit and healthy. His posture showed a marked lumbar lordosis (Fig. 14.8) and examination of his legs showed hypertrophied calf muscles

NEUROLOGICAL DISORDERS 145

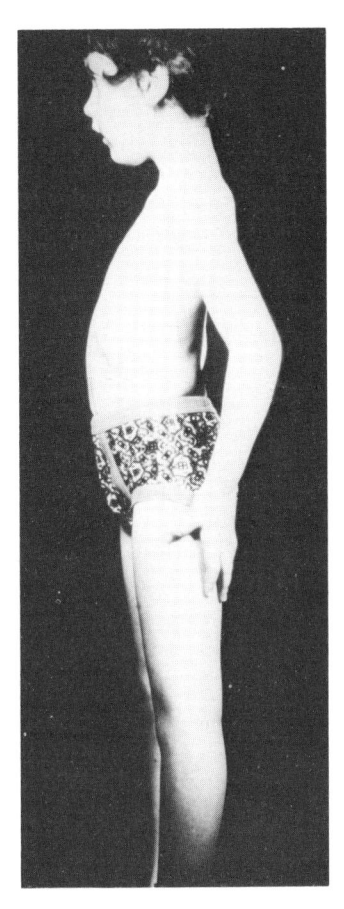

Fig. 14.8
Posture of child with Duchenne muscular dystrophy

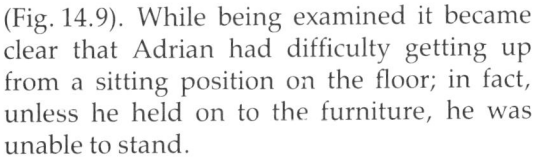

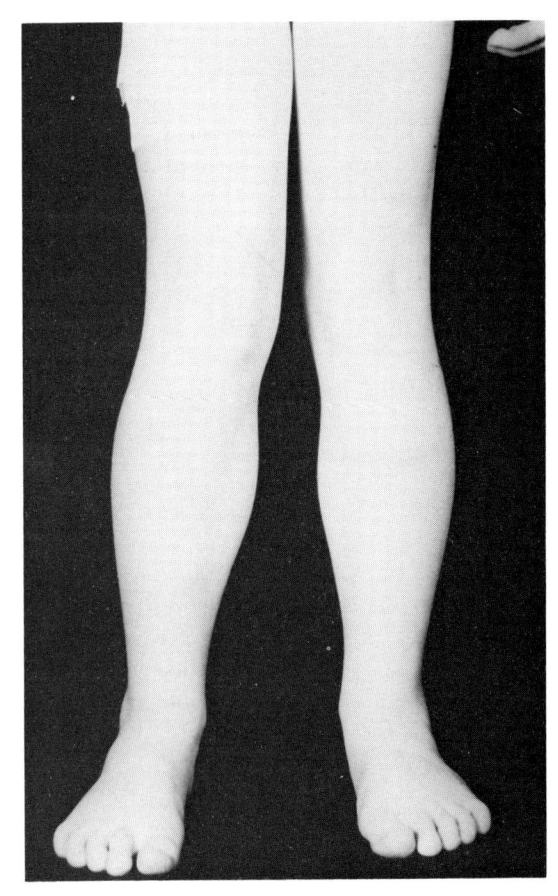

Fig. 14.9
Calf hypertrophy

(Fig. 14.9). While being examined it became clear that Adrian had difficulty getting up from a sitting position on the floor; in fact, unless he held on to the furniture, he was unable to stand.

A clinical diagnosis of Duchenne muscular dystrophy was made. In order to confirm the diagnosis, a serum creatinine phosphokinase level (CPK), electrical studies and muscle biopsy were carried out. A detailed family history was obtained which revealed no other affected members of the family.

Comment

Muscular dystrophies are characterized by slow progressive muscle fibre degeneration. Duchenne is the commonest type, with an incidence of 1 in 4000 births, and is inherited as a sex-linked recessive condition. Early features tend to include a waddling lordotic gait, difficulty in running and a tendency to fall over. Later on, when attempting to get up, the child 'climbs up his legs'—Gowers' sign.

As the disease progresses, most muscle groups are involved but with sparing of facial muscles and hand grip. Hypertrophy is seen in the calf muscles, deltoids, masseter or tongue. Mild intellectual impairment, with an IQ from 70 to 85, is common. Other causes of muscle weakness in children are much less common: the facial muscles are usually involved in myasthenia gravis but the Tensilon (edrophonium) test enables the diagnosis to be made.

Children with Duchenne muscular dystrophy are unable to walk by the age of 8–11, and cannot dress or propel their wheelchair by 13–14 years. Survival ranges from 15 to 25 years, with death commonly occurring from a chest infection or from cardiac failure due to myocardial involvement.

Genetic counselling is indicated once the definitive diagnosis has been made. The mother and her sisters and other daughters will need screening to see if they are carriers of the disease, and CPK measurements are often helpful in finding them. Unfortunately, at present some carriers will remain undetected by such methods and *in utero* diagnosis of Duchenne dystrophy is not yet possible. Clearly, aborting all male fetuses is not a very satisfactory method of prevention.

Blindness

Sally is now 2 years old. She was a second child born at term after an uneventful pregnancy and had a birth weight of 3.50 kg. Although she smiled at 8 weeks, her eyes never seemed to focus on anything and they made continuous roving movements. At 12 weeks she was seen by an ophthalmologist who found a coarse nystagmus and noted that she did not blink or turn away from a bright light shone in her eyes; furthermore she did not fix on objects and follow them.

Her pupils were therefore dilated and her fundi inspected under sedation. The optic discs were small and pale and there was extensive chorioretinitis but a congenital infection screen was negative. Her hearing was intact, so the parents were encouraged to use tactile and vocal stimulation with toys which made noises. Armbands with bells were used in an attempt to teach spatial orientation of the environment.

As she became older it was clear that she could perceive bright lights close to her eyes and sometimes held large bricks close to her face. Motor milestones were only slightly delayed and speech and social skills developed normally. Referral to a toy library was arranged at 15 months, with admission to a special nursery group for visually handicapped children at 20 months. The parents kept in close contact with the Royal National Institute for the Blind, who discussed with them the need for special education in the future.

Comment

Approximately 500 children each year are newly registered as blind or partially sighted—an incidence of 1 in 2500 children. About half these children will have additional handicaps in the form of cerebral palsy, mental handicap or deafness. Among those registered as blind, only 5 per cent have no perception of light but for educational purposes a child is defined as blind if he requires education by methods such as Braille which do not involve sight. Those who are partially sighted will be able to use special methods depending on their residual sight.

The aetiology of blindness varies between western countries and the developing world (Table 14.4). There seems to be little scope for prevention in the UK but rubella vaccination, oxygen monitoring in premature infants and genetic counselling will prevent a few cases. In the tropics xerophthalmia due to vitamin A deficiency and infections such as trachoma and measles predominate. They could all, in theory, be prevented or treated.

It is rarely possible to improve the vision of a blind child, except where there are cataracts, but visual function must be carefully assessed in order to plan management. A standard Snellen chart can be used for children with a mental age over 7 years; assessment below this age is more difficult.

Treatment will depend on whether or not another handicap is present. The blind child with multiple handicaps will need considerable attention, and Sunshine Home Nurseries provided by the RNIB may be suitable during infancy. For the visually handicapped child peripatetic teachers in the home are again provided by the RNIB but residential schooling may be necessary to teach Braille. The help and advice of other workers such as occupational therapists may be needed for the modification of a home to make it a safer, more stimulating environment.

Guillain–Barré Syndrome

Craig, a 12 year old, had been feeling rather miserable for a few days and had then developed a persistent headache, with pains in his lower back and arms. His father noted that he was having difficulty walking and telephoned his GP for advice. The doctor came to the house to see Craig and found that he had considerable weakness of his legs, having difficulty standing unaided. Because of his concerns, and knowing that this was a single-parent family, the GP arranged immediate hospital admission.

Table 14.4
Common causes of visual handicap in children

Western countries	Developing countries
Chorioretinal degeneration	Gonococcal eye infection
Congenital cataracts	Trachoma virus infection
Optic atrophy	Measles
Retrolental fibroplasia	Vitamin A deficiency
Eye injuries	

A further review of the history in hospital revealed that Craig had had pins and needles in both feet for several days before the onset of weakness. Examination showed gross muscle weakness of both legs, with no fasciculation or muscle wasting. Generalized hypotonia was found and no tendon reflexes could be elicited from the legs. The arms were less severely involved and Craig was able to sit up in bed and use a knife and fork for his meals. A lumbar puncture showed a normal cerebrospinal fluid (CSF) pressure, with no increase in cells but with a moderately raised protein content. Spinal x-rays were normal.

During the next week in hospital, Craig's condition rapidly deteriorated with increasing weakness of his trunk muscles and arms which resulted in a complete quadriplegia. Furthermore, there was bilateral facial weakness and some difficulty in swallowing, so nasogastric tube feeding was instituted. There was concern about his respiratory status as he had become cyanosed twice and arterial blood gas analysis showed the following results: pH 7.26, P_{CO_2} 8.3, P_{O_2} 5.4, HCO_3 34, BEx +8; the picture of respiratory failure. He required mechanical ventilation for several days.

After a month Craig's condition improved slowly and he was mobilized during the next two months.

Comment

The term acute inflammatory polyneuropathy is commonly used instead of the eponymous term Guillain–Barré syndrome. Population studies suggest an incidence of 1 in 50 000 of all ages per year, with about two-thirds of cases precipitated by upper respiratory infections. The dorsal and ventral roots of the spinal cord and peripheral nerves show marked degenerative changes and demyelinization. In fact there is evidence of inflammation and degeneration throughout the whole course of the lower motor neuron. There is a wide spectrum of severity. However, the 20 per cent of children most severely affected will need mechanical ventilation if they develop respiratory paralysis or bulbar palsy.

Diagnosis is usually relatively easy with the clinical picture of sudden-onset weakness of all limbs which predominantly involves the proximal muscles and sometimes ascends from legs to arms. Sensory manifestations are much less marked than motor features, and alternative diagnoses such as spinal cord tumour or polio should be easy to refute (Fig. 14.10).

COMMON FEATURES OF GUILLAIN-BARRÉ SYNDROME

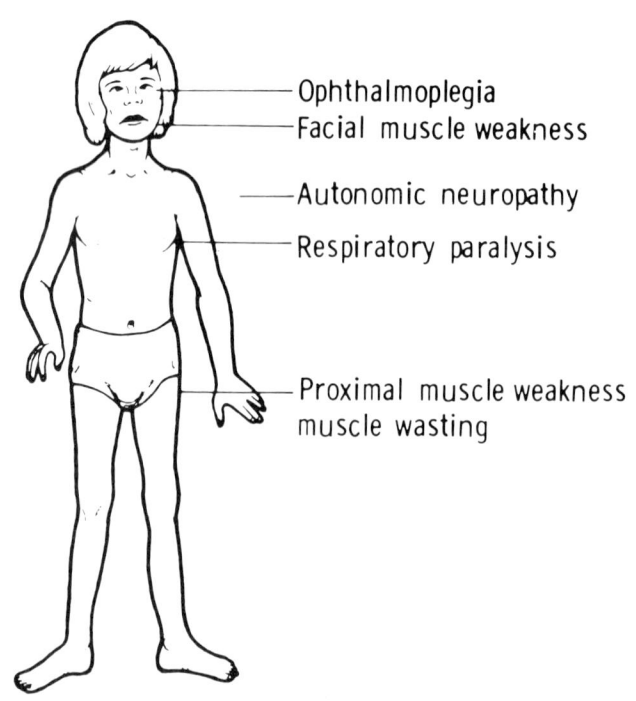

- Ophthalmoplegia
- Facial muscle weakness
- Autonomic neuropathy
- Respiratory paralysis
- Proximal muscle weakness muscle wasting

Fig. 14.10

Features of Guillain–Barré syndrome

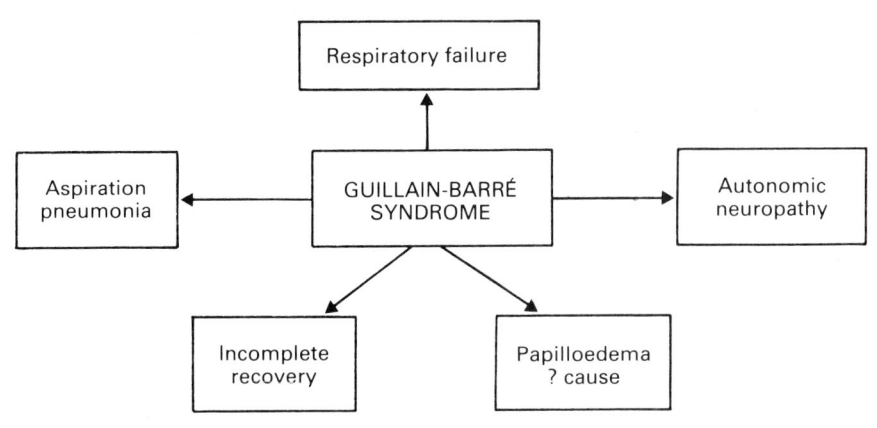

Fig. 14.11
Complications of Gullain–Barré syndrome

No specific treatment alters the course of the disease, and recent trials of steroids have shown adverse effects. Complications do occur (Fig. 14.11) and the occasional death results, usually from respiratory failure. For mobilization and rehabilitation, close liaison with physiotherapists, occupational therapists and hospital teachers is essential because intellectual function is not impaired and psychological support will be needed in an attempt to produce full recovery.

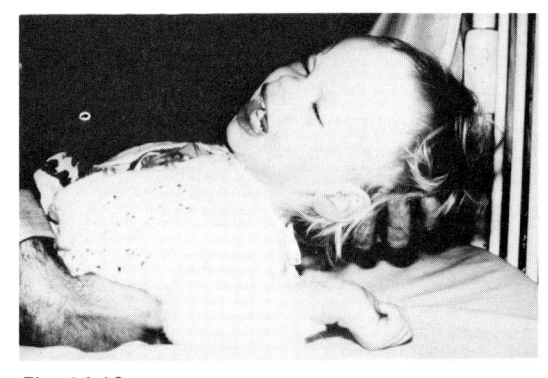

Fig. 14.12
Neck flexion in child with meningitis

Meningitis

Clare, aged 20 months, was admitted to hospital with an eight-hour history of fever and irritability. She had refused to drink anything during this time and became drowsy prior to her admission. Her temperature was found to be 39.4°C; there was marked neck stiffness so that neck flexion was impossible (Fig. 14.12); she was unable to kiss her knees and Kernig's sign was positive (Fig. 14.13). She was drowsy, irritable and not fully aware of the people around her.

A lumbar puncture revealed hazy CSF, which was Gram stained and inspected under

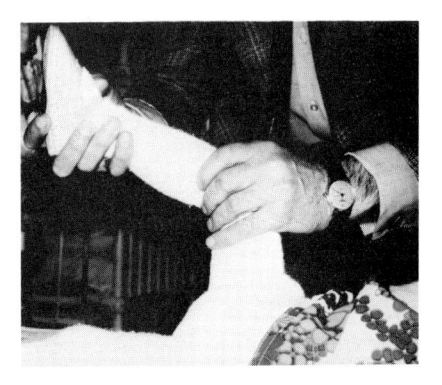

Fig. 14.13
Kernig's sign

the microscope. Gram-negative rods were seen. Nose and throat swabs as well as blood cultures were taken, and antibiotic treatment with intravenous chloramphenicol was commenced. The next day the organisms from the CSF were grown and confirmed to be *Haemophilus influenzae*, which was resistant to ampicillin but sensitive to chloramphenicol. After a week the antibiotics were given orally and discontinued at 12 days. At outpatient review several weeks later, Clare was developmentally and neurologically normal with a normal head size.

Comment

Meningitis is a relatively common infection in children and nearly always presents with signs of systemic illness and meningeal irritation. Diagnosis can sometimes be difficult in 'partially treated' children who have been on antibiotics for treatment of a fever! Occasionally the physical signs will assist in the diagnosis of the specific pathogen involved—an enlarged parotid will suggest mumps, whereas a widespread purpuric rash is likely to be due to a meningococcal infection. Lumbar puncture, which can be preceded by intravenous mannitol when there are signs of raised intracranial pressure, gives a definitive diagnosis and should enable viral and bacterial infections to be distinguished (Table 14.5). Unfortunately the partially treated case may cause confusion, as no organisms will be present on Gram stain and culture will be negative.

In children purulent meningitis is usually caused by Haemophilus, Pneumococcus or Meningococcus but the newborn infant is more likely to have a coliform or group B streptococcal infection. The route of infection is probably via the nasopharynx or middle ear.

Initial treatment of meningitis involves the use of an antibiotic likely to cover most types of organism until CSF culture and sensitivity results are available. High dose ampicillin alone has been superseded by chloramphenicol, as more than 20 per cent of Haemophilus bacteria now produce beta-lactamase. When typical clinical and CSF findings of meningococcal meningitis are present, high dose intravenous penicillin G (300 mg/kg per day) is used. Antibiotics may need modifying at 24–48 hours when further information is available. Viral meningitis will not require specific treatment.

Most children make a full recovery from meningitis (except neonates) but neurological sequelae are found in a few cases. Formal hearing testing after a few months is generally carried out because auditory nerve damage can occur. Long-term follow-up should not be necessary in the majority of children.

Table 14.5

Differences between the three different types of meningitis

	Onset	Lethargy	CSF cells	CSF sugar	Organism on Gram-stained smear
Bacterial	Acute	Present	Polymorphs	Decreased	Usually present
Viral	Acute	Absent	Lymphocytes	Normal	Absent
TB	Subacute	Present	Lymphocytes	Decreased	Absent

Febrile Convulsion

Judy, aged 12 months, was brought to the accident and emergency department at 1:00 a.m., having had a generalized convulsion lasting about 20 minutes. The fit stopped spontaneously in the ambulance just before arrival at the hospital.

She had apparently been well until 12 hours before when her mother said she became miserable, felt hot and was off her food. As she was unwell she slept in her parents' bed but suddenly awoke, cried out, and became rigid with generalized shaking movements of both arms and legs. Her breathing was noisy and she did not recognize her mother. Her father thought she was about to die and 'phoned 999 for an ambulance. The ambulancemen found Judy cyanosed on their arrival at the house and administered oxygen by facemask en route to the hospital.

The casualty officer noted that there was no family history of convulsions and that there had been no previous similar episodes. The child was hot to touch and had a temperature of 39°C, with no localized sign of infection other than a red pharynx. Although sleepy on arrival, she woke up over the next half hour and had no localized neurological signs. Her capillary blood glucose was checked with a BM-Test Glycemie 20–800 stick and found to be 5 mmol/l. A lumbar puncture was performed since meningitis may present in this way, even in the absence of meningeal signs.

Comment

Judy had had a febrile convulsion, a grand mal convulsion with a fever which happens to 3 per cent of young children. They are rare under 6 months and over 5 years of age (Fig. 14.14). The overall chance of recurrent febrile convulsions is about 1 in 3. Very few children (about 1 per cent) with febrile convulsions go on to have epilepsy in childhood. Temporal lobe damage may occasionally be sustained after a prolonged convulsion lasting more than half an hour, and predisposes to temporal lobe epilepsy.

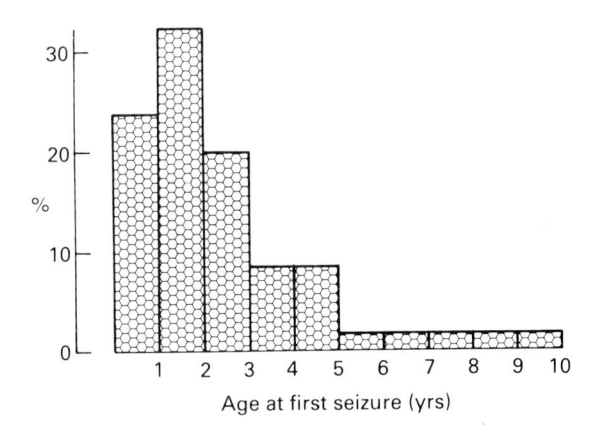

Fig. 14.14

Age distribution of children with febrile fits

Table 14.6

Advice to parents on preventing febrile convulsions

Skin exposure	Undress the child, keep away from the fire or radiator
Enourage fluids	To prevent dehydration
Antipyretic drugs	Paracetamol or aspirin
Tepid sponging	To remove heat by evaporation

Prevention of recurrent fits involves advice to parents on temperature control during intercurrent infection (Table 14.6)—the rate of increase in temperature as well as the peak are important. If the convulsions are repeated or prolonged, prophylactic anticonvulsants are indicated. It is pointless giving a drug such as phenobarbitone at the time of fever as it takes at least a week to achieve adequate brain levels! Phenobarbitone and sodium valproate are equally effective given once daily and up to 70 per cent of fits may be prevented, although behavioural problems occur with the former.

In the child who has fits in spite of these measures, rectal diazepam given by the parents may be helpful. The prognosis for the vast majority of children with febrile fits is excellent—nearly all disappear by 7 years of age, and sequelae are rare.

Cerebral Palsy

Paul, a 20 month old, was seen by the family doctor at the weekly child health clinic because of his mother's concern about his gait. The pregnancy had been uneventful and went to term but there was fetal distress during the latter part of the labour which necessitated an emergency caesarean section. The baby was asphyxiated at birth and needed resuscitation until spontaneous breathing was established at 12 minutes.

An initial glance at the child revealed an unusual posture of the left arm which was abducted at the shoulder and flexed at the elbow. It did not swing during walking. The gait was abnormal, with less movement on the left side and persistent plantar flexion of the foot when the leg was lifted. Hypertonia and increased reflexes were present on the left side—the findings of a spastic hemiplegia. The social and language skills appeared relatively preserved. After discussion with the mother a second opinion was sought. The findings were confirmed without any other evidence of handicap. Regular physiotherapy was commenced with the use of passive and active movements in an effort to reduce the muscle contracture. Progress was reasonable and three years later the abnormal gait was less obvious.

Comment

Cerebral palsy is a disorder present in 2 per 1000 children. It is defined as a permanent non-progressive brain abnormality occurring in early life and producing disordered motor function. There is a high incidence of associated problems due to more widespread cerebral dysfunction (Table 14.7). The average IQ is 70, with 74 per cent having a quotient less

Table 14.7

Associations with cerebral palsy

Mental retardation
Epilepsy
Squint
Speech disorders
Visual impairment
Hearing loss
Perceptual defects
Behaviour problems

Table 14.8

Causes of cerebral palsy

Cerebral malformations
Hypoxia
Trauma (accidental and non-accidental)
Kernicterus
Hypoglycaemia
CNS infection
Vascular accidents
Poisoning

than 90. Emotional disorders are common and educational difficulties may be more severe than expected because of subtle perceptual difficulties.

The aetiology is known in about half of all cases (Table 14.8) and the disorder is classified by the type of motor disorder (spastic, hypotonic or athetoid) and according to the functional deficit (Fig. 14.15). Spastic hemiplegia makes up approximately one-third of all cases (Fig. 14.16).

The time of presentation of cerebral palsy depends on its severity. Many cases will present because of delayed motor milestones.

Early diagnosis is important as there is evidence accumulating of the benefit of early physiotherapy techniques such as Bobath's, which utilize motor responses to posture changes, to evoke active movements in the

Hemiplegia   Quadriplegia   Diplegia

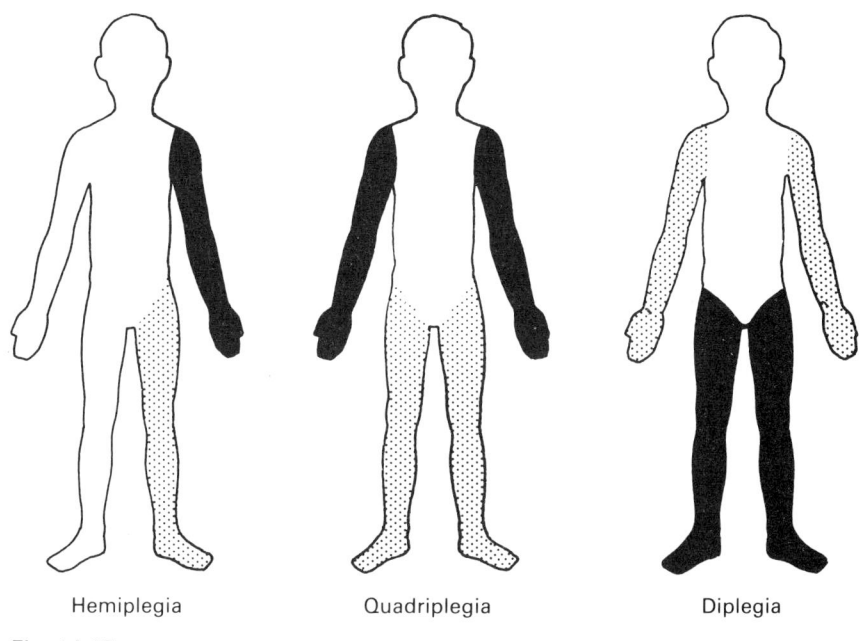

Fig. 14.15
Types of spastic cerebral palsy

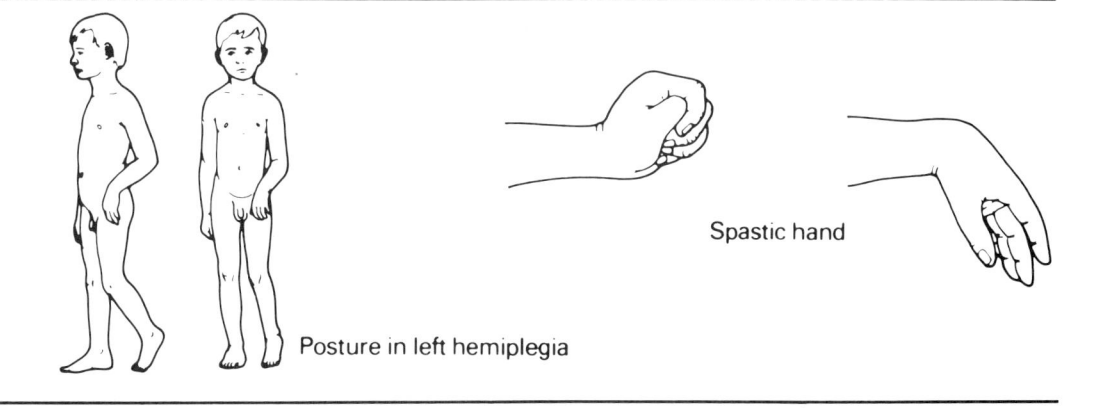

Posture in left hemiplegia

Spastic hand

Fig. 14.16
Features of hemiplegia

child who is too young to give conscious cooperation. Physiotherapy is not very helpful for severe athetoid cerebral palsy.

Clearly the aims of treatment must be to maximize the handicapped child's potential. A 'cure' is not possible but mild or moderate hemiplegias without any other deficit can sometimes leave few residual problems when the child is grown up. The more severe forms of cerebral palsy such as spastic quadriplegia will need more intensive management and their outlook will not be so good.

Migraine

Andrew, an 8-year-old child of West Indian parents, developed episodes of vomiting which lasted about 24 hours before they suddenly disappeared spontaneously. During these episodes he would develop a headache, become pale and listless, and rub and squeeze his eyes as if they hurt. Andrew had missed many days off school because of these attacks which seemed to arrive twice a week, without obvious precipitating cause. When a careful history was taken it became clear that Andrew's mother developed classic attacks of migraine as a teenager and that she still tended to have these premenstrually.

A full examination, which included a check of blood pressure, optic fundi and the nervous system, was normal, and there was no intracranial bruit. Migraine was diagnosed and specific enquiry was made about visual aura. Andrew was not able to add anything other than saying his head hurt but when given a crayon and paper he was able to draw a picture of what he saw when he was rubbing his eyes.

At this initial assessment the parents were asked to make a note of food intake during the 24 hours prior to the attacks, in an attempt to elucidate whether any specific foods such as chocolate, cheese, Marmite or specific fruits precipitated attacks. It was suggested that aspirin or paracetamol be given early in the attack. The attacks often followed eating oranges.

Comment

Migraine is a common cause of headache in children. About 4 per cent of children under 10 years suffer from migraine, but few are actually diagnosed in practice. The first clue is a positive family history, which is present in 80 per cent of cases. Most commonly the first sign of an attack is headache affecting one side of the head. Sometimes direct questioning early in an attack will reveal paraesthesia in the extremities. Clearly the description of symptoms is age dependent, so diagnosis may be difficult in young children. Descriptions of visual aura should be specifically asked for; comments like 'I can see fireworks' or 'Everything looks funny' alert one to the presence of a visual aura.

Investigations of migrainous headaches for a treatable organic lesion is necessary only in certain circumstances, listed in Table 14.9.

Table 14.9

Migraine should be investigated

When there are focal neurological signs
When there is a cranial bruit
When there are signs of raised intracranial pressure
When the headaches are becoming more severe and more frequent

When any of these features is present then alternative diagnosis such as arteriovenous malformation or brain tumour should be considered, and further investigation arranged.

Treatment involves removal of trigger factors such as foods high in tyramine or other amines or chemical neurotransmitters, and reduction of intervals between meals or stress factors. Often aspirin or paracetamol are adequate treatment if given early in an attack but some children will need non-ergotamine migraine therapy. Fortunately, many children will lose their migraine attacks at puberty.

15 Miscellaneous

Obesity

Barrington was an 11-year-old boy whose problem was obesity. His class teacher had become increasingly worried about his withdrawn behaviour, which was felt to be a direct result of his excessive weight. He was referred to hospital by the school doctor.

He was born in Jamaica and moved to England when he was 3 years old. He was bottle fed from birth and cereals were started when he was only 6 weeks old. His mother had no record of weights in infancy but said that he had always been a big baby and a big child. She didn't think that he ate excessively and didn't seem worried that he was overweight. A dietitian assessed Barrington's diet and calculated that his daily intake was about 3500 calories. Further questioning revealed that he was constantly being teased at school, often very cruelly. He had become progressively very solitary and withdrawn, rarely mixing with other children.

Table 15.1

Health consequences of obesity in adults

Reduced life expectancy
Higher incidence of atherosclerosis
Higher incidence of chronic bronchitis
Higher incidence of spinal and hip degenerative disease
Increased risk of accidents
Higher life insurance premiums

On examination he was obviously obese. His weight and height were measured and plotted on a percentile chart, together with previous recordings made at school (Figs. 15.1 and 15.2). Note that he is tall for age and that his height and weight are out of proportion.

The doctor examining Barrington noted with dismay that his mother was enormous, as was the baby she was holding in her arms.

Comment

Obesity is the commonest nutritional disorder of children in the western world. There is good evidence that many fat children become fat adults. Obesity is unhealthy (Table 15.1).

Obesity is a condition in which the whole adipose organ is enlarged out of proportion to other body tissues. It can be assessed in a number of ways. Body weight, plotted on a percentile chart, gives an indication of the 'normality' of a particular child's weight (compared with supposedly normal children). Naturally, height affects weight and this can be allowed for. Thickness of subcutaneous fat can be simply measured using skinfold calipers, and percentile charts give the range of thickness at different ages. In practice, simple observation of the undressed child leaves little doubt about the diagnosis.

The incidence is difficult to define but at least 3 per cent of British school children are obese. The cause of obesity is an energy intake in excess of a child's requirements. The excess energy is stored as fat in adipose cells. Whilst

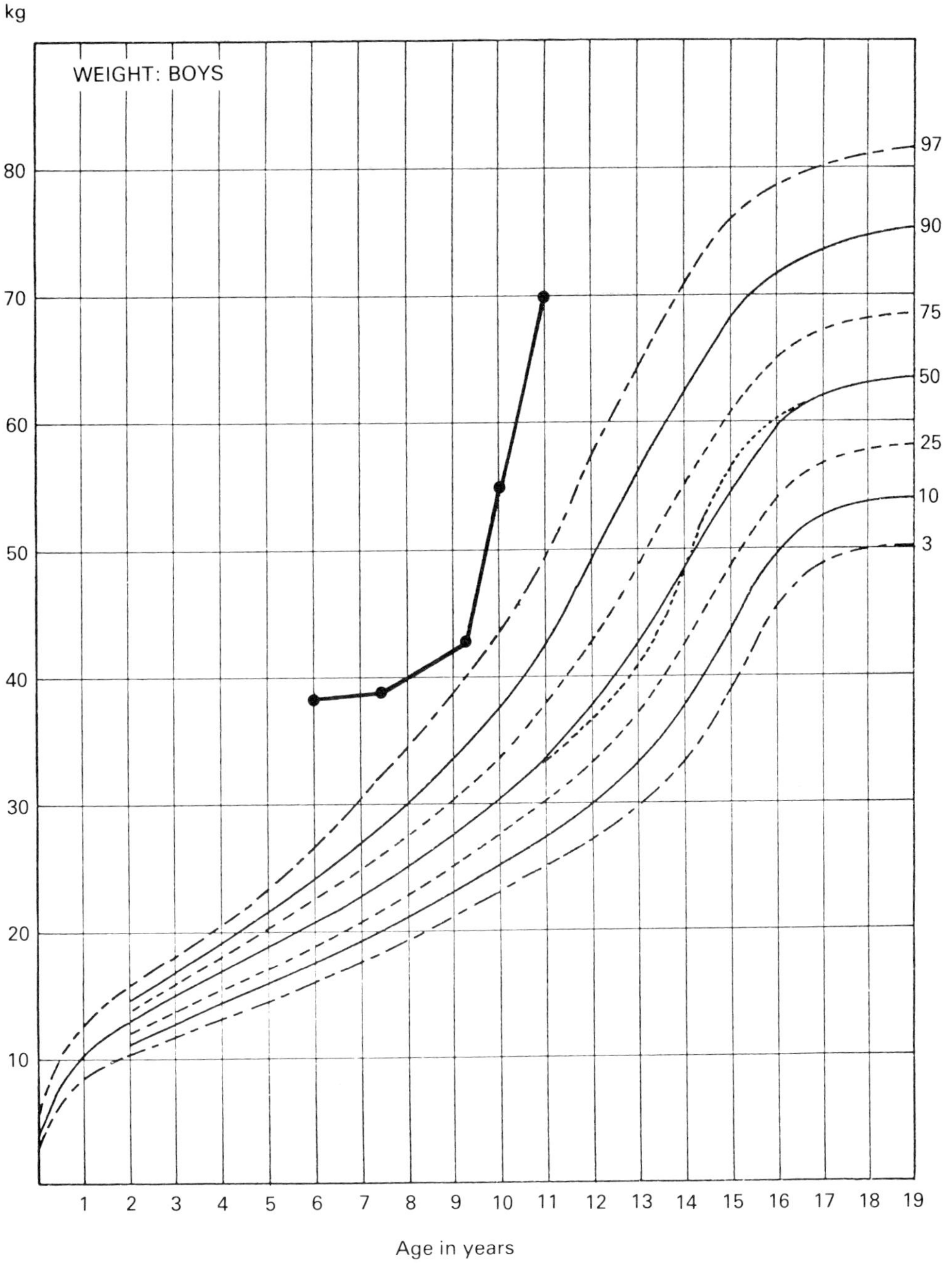

MISCELLANEOUS 157

Fig. 15.1
Weight chart in obesity

158 CLINICAL CASES IN PAEDIATRICS

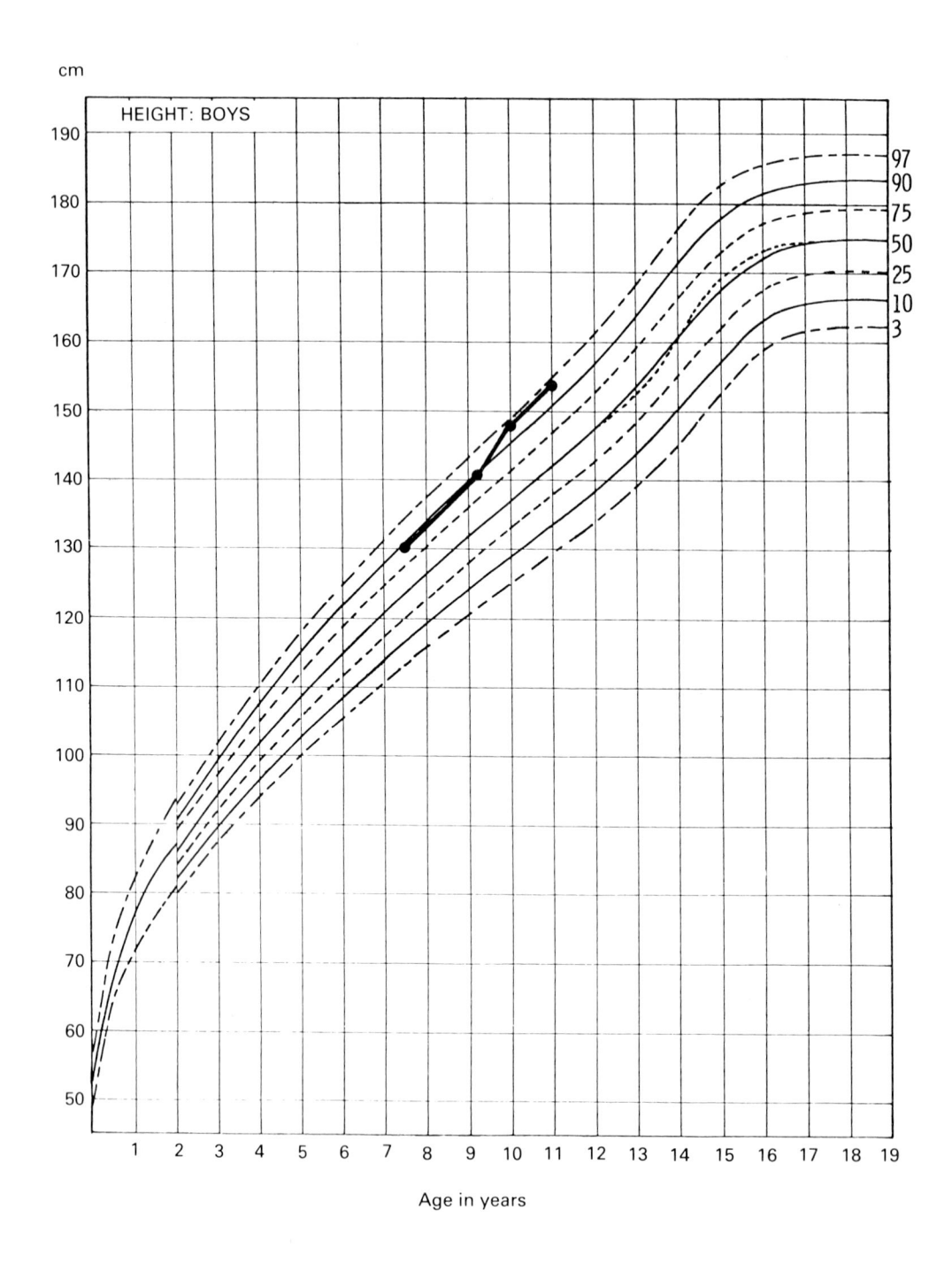

Fig. 15.2
Height chart in obesity

genetic factors play a role in determining obesity, environmental factors are more important. Overeating is the main cause, although it is not known why a particular calorie intake makes one child obese but keeps another child at an appropriate weight. Unhappy children often eat excessively, although it is difficult to separate cause and effect. Energy expenditure is reduced in fat children because of their reluctance to take physical exercise.

The emotional effects of obesity are underestimated. There is still a mistaken idea that fat children are jolly, amiable and tolerant. They are often desperately unhappy and isolated.

Barrington agreed that he was overweight and because he seemed reasonably interested in dieting an 800 kcal reducing diet was recommended. His mother, however, did not appear keen, and compliance was poor. A year later Barrington stopped coming to the clinic.

Prevention is a more worthwhile approach to the problem of obesity and can take the form of advice and education to both the mother and the child.

Chronic Juvenile Arthritis

Philip, a 7 year old, presented with a two-month history of joint pains involving his wrists, hands, knees and feet. His parents thought he had lost some weight during this time and commented that he had had an intermittent fever. When examined, he looked well but there was swelling of the joints with diffuse involvement of interphalangeal joints of the hands, knee effusions with muscle wasting of the thighs and limited abduction of the left hip joint.

Hospital admission was arranged immediately for further investigation and treatment. A mild anaemia was detected, with a neutrophilia and a raised ESR of 55 mm per hour.

The serum IgG level was slightly raised, although levels of other immunoglobulins were normal. Specific tests for rheumatoid and antinuclear factors were negative. X-rays showed some oesteoporosis of the hands, but no specific abnormalities.

Treatment was begun with aspirin given in sufficient doses to maintain therapeutic blood levels, and this resulted in some pain relief. Night splints were used to keep the joints comfortable in a position of rest. Physiotherapists initially helped with passive exercises to build up muscle bulk, and then assisted with mobilization. Swimming seemed to be helpful as Philip was able to exercise without weight bearing. Schooling continued while in hospital, and a peripatetic teacher was arranged for the first few months at home. The parents were able to work closely with physiotherapists and twice-weekly hospital visits were undertaken.

Comment

Philip had juvenile chronic arthritis (Still's disease), which is not a specific disease entity, and he fell in the group of *polyarticular* disease seen in about half such children (Fig. 15.3). Where there are fewer than four joints involved (*pauciarticular* disease) iridocyclitis is likely to occur over a ten-year period and can cause blindness. Such children are commonly girls who have antinuclear factor present in their serum, so regular slit lamp examinations are essential for early detection. The major morbidity of this group lies in the eyes rather than in the joints. HLA typing of boys with pauciarticular disease reveals a high incidence of HLA-B27 haplotype, a group who probably have early ankylosing spondylitis. The systemic form, with fever, rash, lymphadenopathy and splenomegaly, occurs in younger children.

Management of joint disease involves close

co-operation between parents and hospital staff. Aspirin is the most useful anti-inflammatory drug, but may cause gastric upset. There are many other newer, non-steroidal anti-inflammatory agents, which may be tried if aspirin does not work or is not tolerated.

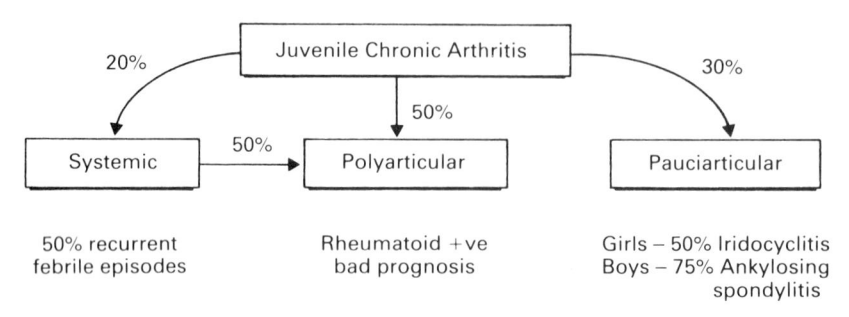

Fig. 15.3
Classification of chronic juvenile arthritis

Steroids are rarely used (Table 15.2) because they stunt growth, which will have already been compromised during the active disease process. The long-term prognosis for Philip is good as only 10 per cent of children with polyarticular disease who are rheumatoid factor negative will develop destructive arthritis and permanent joint deformity.

Table 15.2
Indications for steroid therapy in juvenile chronic polyarthritis

Severe systemic disease
Severe joint disease unresponsive to other measures
Chronic iridocyclitis

Phenylketonuria

Daisy was born at term following a normal pregnancy, labour and delivery. The Guthrie test taken on the sixth day (Fig. 15.4) was abnormal, with a phenylalanine level of 1500 μmol/l (normal < 240 μmol/l). An urgent referral to a paediatrician was therefore arranged. She found a normal infant who had a positive Phenistix urine test. Chromatography of this urine revealed the presence of phenylketones, and plasma amino acid chromatography revealed a high peak of phenylalanine and low tyrosine levels.

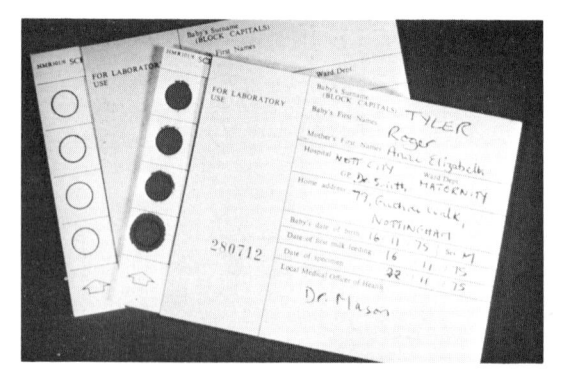

Fig. 15.4
Guthrie test card

It was felt likely that Daisy had classic phenylketonuria (PKU), and a low phenylalanine diet was commenced using Minafen (a protein hydrolysate) with small supplements of cows' milk. A senior dietitian liaised closely with the doctor and she supervised the dietary management and education of the parents. Regular capillary phenylalanine levels were monitored, aiming to keep levels between 250 and 500 µmol/l. The diet was difficult to administer because of the unpalatable nature of the protein hydrolysates.

A challenge at six months produced very high phenylalanine levels again, so the disease did not appear to be a transient phenomenon. Regular developmental assessments showed normal progress during the first few years.

Comment

PKU has an incidence of 1 in 10 000 births in the UK. Screening using urine tests is unreliable, and a national screening programme using capillary blood on the Guthrie test (which is a microbiological assay) was introduced in 1969. There is a deficiency of the enzyme phenylalanine hydroxylase which converts phenylalanine to tyrosine (Fig. 15.5). Because of the metabolic block, excessive phenylketones are produced, and these spill over into the urine which is often positive on Phenistix or ferric chloride testing (Fig. 15.6). Inheritance is recessive, so the parents can be assumed to be asymptomatic carriers.

Untreated children who were diagnosed late before the advent of mass screening were severely mentally retarded, with developmental quotients around 30. They tended to have hyperactivity, with aggressive behaviour, and their response to late treatment was poor. Now that diagnosis can be made at a few weeks of age, treatment can be instituted at an early stage to prevent the high phenylalanine levels which produce this cerebral

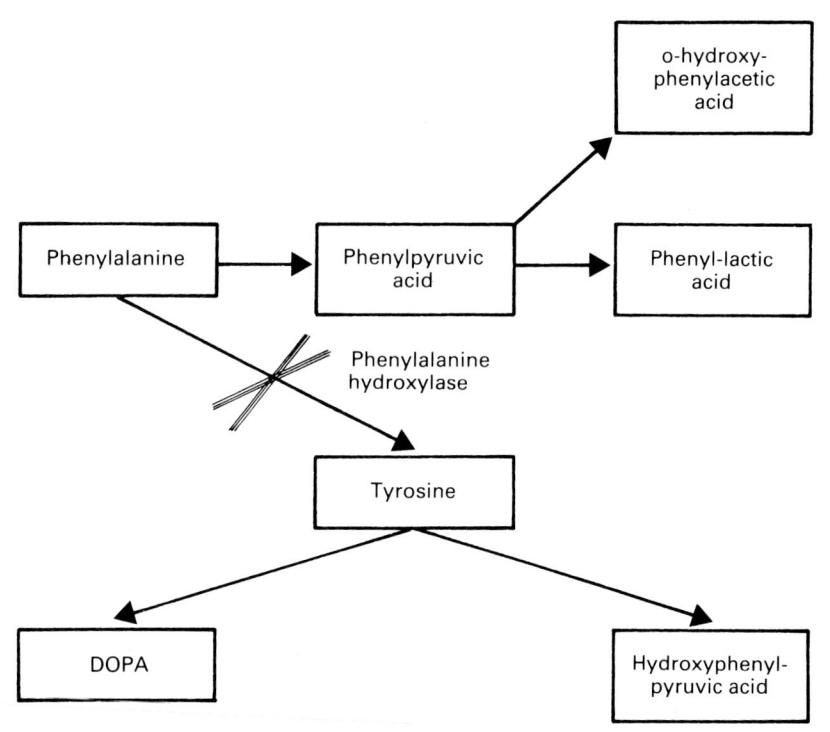

Fig. 15.5
Site of metabolic block in phenylketonuria

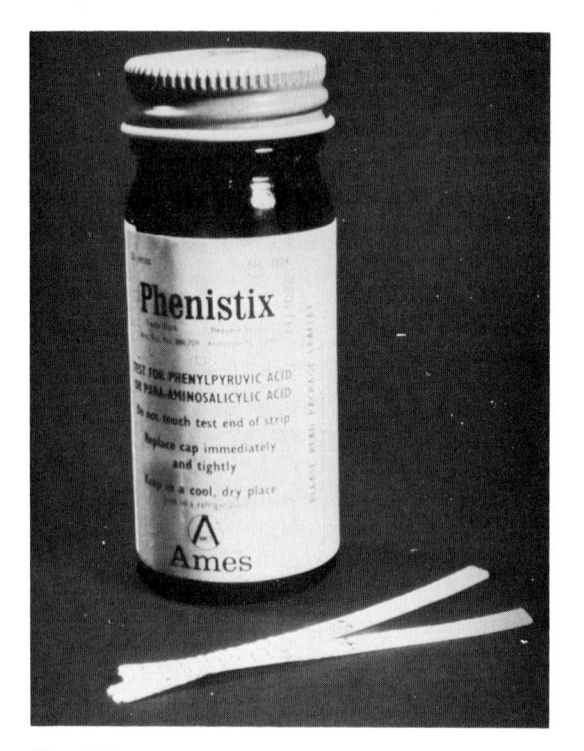

Fig. 15.6
Phenistix strips

damage. The difficulty with the dietary management is administering sufficient phenylalanine, which is an essential amino acid, to produce growth without giving toxic blood levels. Clearly, feeding a toddler an unpleasant diet will be difficult, and intercurrent infections make problems more difficult by causing breakdown of endogenous protein and increasing phenylalanine levels.

The diet is usually relaxed by about 8 years of age to maintain phenylalanine levels below 1000 μmol/l, but careful checks of intellectual performance will be needed to ensure that all is well. Attention has recently been directed at maternal PKU during pregnancy. It appears that strict dietary measures are needed from the time of conception to prevent fetal damage by high maternal phenylalanine concentrations.

The results of treatment of this classic metabolic disease are good in spite of the practical dietary difficulties during the first few years of life.

Rickets

Sundip, a 3-year-old child of Asian parents, had been unwell for several months with rather vague symptoms such as poor appetite and tiredness. When his mother took him out shopping he refused to walk more than a few yards before wanting to use the pushchair, whereas he had previously been able to walk several hundred yards. He had been seen several times by doctors who could not find any specific abnormality. His mother knew her health visitor quite well, so she took Sundip to the local child health clinic for a further review.

The clinic doctor found Sundip to be a small child who looked pale. His gait was wobbly and he had very marked bow legs, which had apparently been painful at times. Both wrists were tender and swollen, but there were no signs of arthritis. An x-ray of his right wrist revealed the cause of the swelling as rickets (Fig. 15.7). The abnormalities are described in Fig. 15.8. The blood count revealed a mild iron deficiency anaemia with a Hb of 9.6 g/dl, and the biochemical investigations confirmed the clinical and radiological appearances of rickets (Table 15.3). No further investigations were carried out and Sundip was commenced on oral iron and vitamin D therapy.

At review six weeks later, his anaemia had disappeared, and he was just beginning to become more mobile. The wrist swelling was much less obvious. In view of his pathological bow legging an orthopaedic opinion was arranged, but it was decided to wait and see whether corrective osteotomies to the legs could be avoided. It was felt that vitamin D treatment alone would probably result in dra-

MISCELLANEOUS **163**

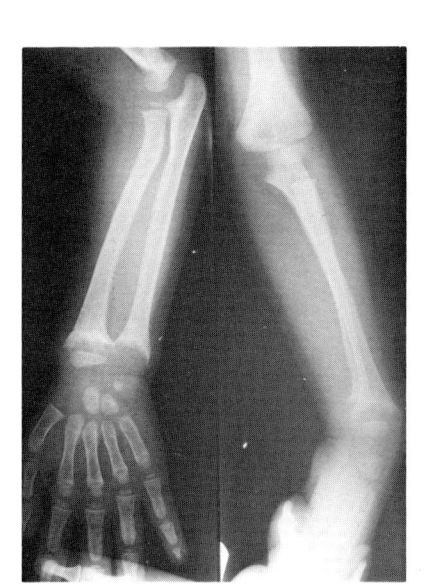

Fig. 15.7
X-ray of rickets

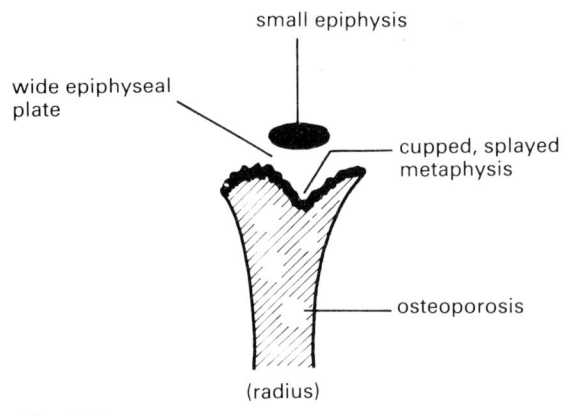

Fig. 15.8
Radiological appearances in rickets

Table 15.3
Biochemical investigations in a child with nutritional rickets

Serum calcium	2.2 mmol/l (normal 2.2–2.6)
Serum phosphate	0.7 mmol/l (normal 1.1–1.8)
Alkaline phosphatase	700 IU/l (normal 70–200)

Urea and electrolytes are normal

matic improvement and surgery would be unnecessary.

Comment

Rickets is a disease of growing bones related to lack of vitamin D. Nutritional rickets is by far the commonest type, tending to occur at times of maximal growth; that is, in premature babies, infants and adolescents. Asian children are especially prone to the disease because of poor skin production of vitamin D from ultraviolet light and inadequate intake on a vegetarian diet (Fig. 15.9). Adolescent rickets is seen only in Asian girls. Osteomalacia can occur during pregnancy, a time when vitamin D and calcium requirements are high, so the baby can develop neonatal rickets. Vitamin D supplements should be given to pregnant Asian mothers.

There are numerous clinical features of rickets such as craniotabes (ping-pong ball skull), frontal bossing of the skull and a 'rickety rosary' due to swelling of the rib costochondral junctions. Knock knees seem to occur only in adolescent rickets. Other members of the family should be screened when an index case is identified, looking for iron deficiency anaemia and biochemical evidence of vitamin D deficiency.

Prevention of rickets could be achieved by health education at a local and national level. Chapatti flour should be supplemented with vitamin D, as are many foodstuffs, but the DHSS has been vacillating about this for many years. Specific information by leaflet or video will need to be provided in the appropriate dialect for the local Asian community. A greater input of time and resources is needed

164 CLINICAL CASES IN PAEDIATRICS

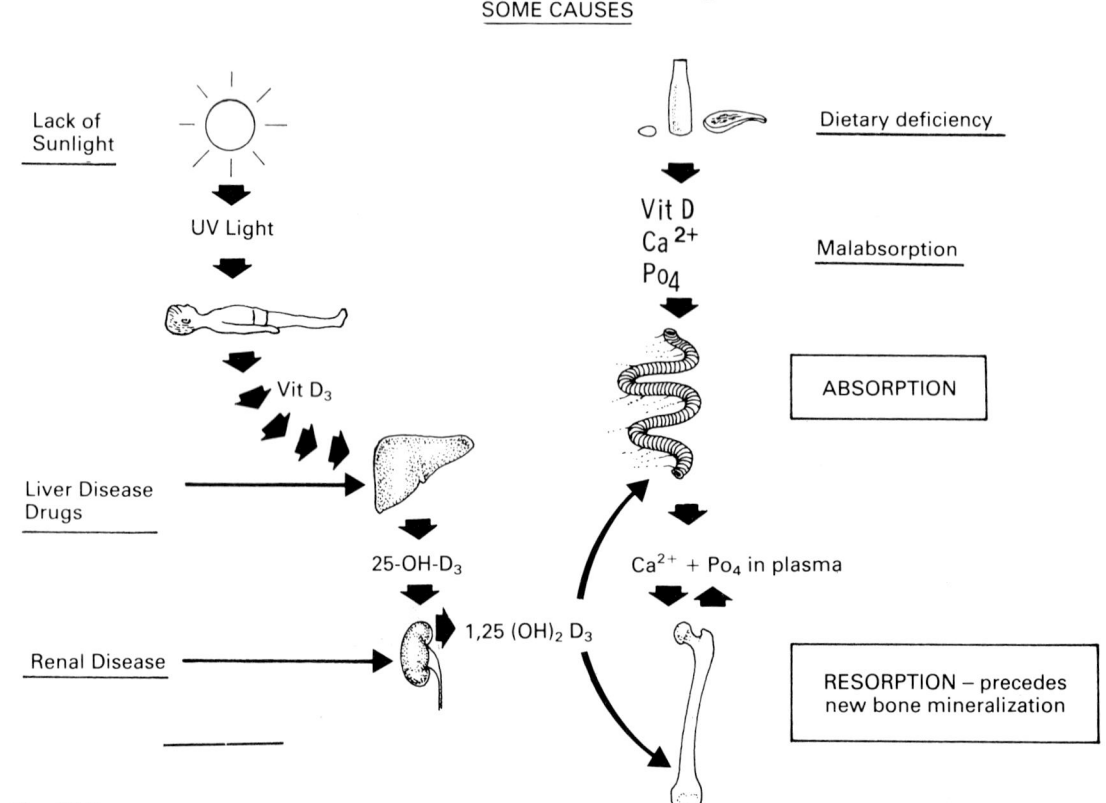

RICKETS
Inadequate Mineralization of Growing Bone
SOME CAUSES

Lack of Sunlight

UV Light

Vit D$_3$

Liver Disease
Drugs

25-OH-D$_3$

Renal Disease

1,25 (OH)$_2$ D$_3$

Dietary deficiency

Vit D
Ca^{2+}
P$_{O_4}$

Malabsorption

ABSORPTION

Ca^{2+} + P$_{O_4}$ in plasma

RESORPTION – precedes new bone mineralization

Fig. 15.9
Biochemistry of rickets

for the prevention of this disease which is difficult to diagnose in its early stages and has a high morbidity.

Cot Death

Mrs C was a 40-year-old mother with two grown-up children. She became unexpectedly pregnant again and delivered twin girls at 35 weeks by dates. The first born, Susan, was a normal delivery, weighing 1.90 kg; the second twin, Janet, was a normal delivery, weighing 1.85 kg. Both babies were transferred to the special care baby unit after birth because of low birth weight. They both became mildly jaundiced in the first week, but had no serious neonatal illnesses. They were both bottle fed and by the twelfth day they were feeding well enough to be discharged. The parents, having got over the surprise of having two babies at their age, were delighted with them.

At home the twins made excellent progress. They were seen regularly at their child health clinic by the health visitor and clinical medical officer, who were pleased that they were thriving and developing normally.

When the twins were 5 months old, they both developed colds and were off colour.

Susan, in particular, was fretful and anorexic, and her mother nursed her until the early hours of the morning when she went to sleep. The following morning she appeared lively and recovered. She was given a bottle of milk but because she still seemed a bit fretful, she was put down in her cot again, lying on her side. An hour later, her mother found her face down in the cot, blue in the face, with milk coming from the corner of her mouth. She was dead, and attempts at artificial respiration were unsuccessful (her family doctor arrived within a few minutes).

normally be expected to kill a child. Numerous explanations have been put forward to explain the deaths, including allergy, overwhelming viral infection and suffocation. The age distribution of cot death shows a peak at 3 months of age (Fig. 15.10). Cot deaths make up a substantial part of the infant mortality figures, which have fallen rapidly in countries such as Holland and Finland but more slowly in the UK.

A coroner's post-mortem was carried out on Susan. The pathologist noted that she was well nourished and well cared for, with no

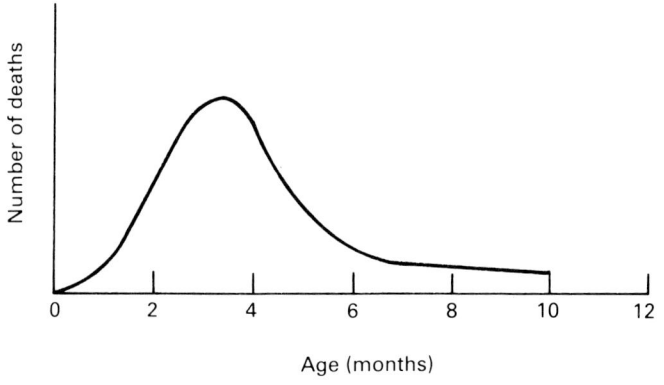

Fig. 15.10
Age distribution of cot death

Comment

The sudden infant death syndrome (SIDS) or cot death are terms used to describe deaths such as this one. A child, usually in the first year of life, having been previously healthy, develops a minor condition such as diarrhoea, vomiting or an upper respiratory infection from which the parents fully expect him to recover. There are 1500 such deaths each year in the UK, and these can even occur in hospital when a child has been admitted for routine surgery or with minor symptoms. The post-mortem finding may show an abnormality such as bronchitis or otitis, which would not

signs of injury. The nose, mouth and trachea contained milk. The mucosa of the bronchi was reddened and the lungs showed areas of consolidation. Microscopy showed evidence of acute infection of the bronchi and lungs. The cause of death was given as an acute, overwhelming respiratory infection—it was thought that the milk in the trachea was a result of terminal inhalation and not the primary cause of death.

Janet recovered from her cold without difficulty and is very well. Her parents were naturally very distressed about Susan's death, in particular because the cause of death was found to be an infection when they had not thought that she was particularly ill and had not sought medical advice. They were terrified that the same thing might happen to Janet. Janet and the parents were seen by the paediatrician, who explained the phenomenon of cot deaths, emphasizing that the parents were in no way to blame for what had happened. He also took the opportunity to examine Janet carefully and reassure them that she was a healthy girl.

Food Intolerance

Rona, a 1-year-old only child, was seen at the request of her mother, who wanted advice on the management of her 'food allergies'. During the previous few months she had developed mild eczema, which was partially controlled with topical steroid treatment. Her mother had noted a further improvement following replacement of cows' milk with a soya milk preparation. There were numerous other concerns about her health, which mainly centred around vomiting and slow growth. The father, a wealthy property speculator, was not very involved in the dietary manipulations and felt that at least it gave his wife something to do at home.

A few weeks before being seen in outpatients, Rona's mother had removed all meat, poultry, eggs and other dairy products from her diet. In coming to these decisions the mother had sought advice from a number of friends and professionals, including two doctors, a dietitian and the local health food shop. The home was littered with books and magazines on food allergy, which enabled the mother to quote articles and references in her discussions about Rona. During the course of the interview an early feeding history was taken and it became clear that there were guilt feelings about her failure to breast feed, as she knew that this afforded some protection against the later development of eczema.

The consultation proved difficult because of the preconceived ideas of the mother combined with an inflexible approach. An element of manipulation was apparent, with one professional being played off against another. Rona's mother wanted the paediatrician to withdraw sucrose and all food additives from her diet, and when this suggestion met with little enthusiasm, she picked Rona up and stormed out of the clinic.

Comment

Food sensitivity is an emotive area and there is a wide range of current attitudes to the subject, depending on whether one is an academic immunologist or an allergist in private practice. The spectrum of views ranges from those who deny its existence to others who attribute a wide range of symptoms to food sensitivity. Unfortunately at present there is a lack of a specific diagnostic test, so the diagnosis of food allergy is largely based on accurate history taking. It is thought that the incidence of food sensitivity is around 2 per cent in western countries; many of these cases are relatively minor, easily recognized by the parents and treated without help from a doctor.

A more common situation is one where the child has been placed on a special diet by the parents, perhaps substituting goats' milk or soya milk for cows' milk or removing (or attempting to remove) all animal proteins. This seems to be particularly common in higher income families.

In practice, the easiest way to resolve the situation when the history is suggestive of food sensitivity is to challenge the child with the food on three occasions. A return of symptoms should be virtually diagnostic. In some situations such as egg allergy, which is relatively common, angioneurotic oedema of the face tends to develop and such challenges are not justified. Hospital admission is advisable where there is the risk of severe reactions such as in a few cases of cows' milk protein intolerance.

Most children with food sensitivity are less than 2 years old, and the manifestations commonly seen are listed in Table 15.4. The most

Table 15.4
Symptoms of food intolerance

Vomiting	47%
Diarrhoea	41%
Crying, 'colicky'	35%
Failure to thrive	31%
Eczema	22%
Abdominal pain	19%
Wheezing	19%
Urticaria	18%

common foods involved are eggs, milk, wheat, chicken or fish. When symptoms are severe and food sensitivity is likely, a basic elimination diet can be given for two or three weeks (Table 15.5) and foods slowly reintroduced at weekly intervals. It is an extremely severe diet. Laboratory tests such as jejunal biopsy help exclude coeliac disease and may help in the diagnosis of cows' milk intolerance. Specific IgE measurements against particular antigens using a radioallergosorbent technique (RAST) on rare occasions provide

Table 15.5
An elimination diet for severe allergic symptoms

Exclude the following:
Beef, pork, poultry
Wheat, rye, oats, barley, corn
Vegetables (except carrots)
Fruit (except pears, peaches, apricots)
Coffee, squashes, Oxo, Bovril
Eggs, fish
Cows' milk and all other dairy products

helpful information to support a diagnosis of a specific food allergy.

It is generally agreed that treatment involves dietary avoidance, with advice from a skilled dietitian rather than drug treatment with oral steroids, disodium cromoglycate or ketotifen. Many of these food sensitivities appear to be a temporary phenomenon which spontaneously resolves once the child is over 2 years.

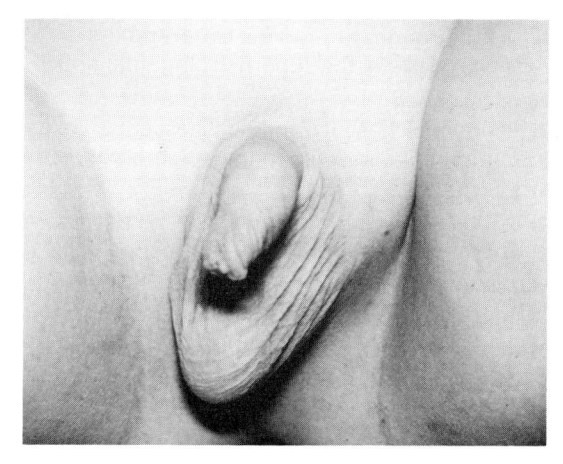

Fig. 15.11
Left undescended testis

Undescended Testes

Justin was seen two days after his first birthday for a routine check at his child health clinic. He had just recovered from whooping cough, and his health visitor arranged this visit as Justin had not previously attended and had received no routine immunizations.

The examination was normal except that the left testis could not be felt although his genitalia were otherwise normal (Fig. 15.11). Justin's mother had never seen his testes, even in the bath! He had recovered his weight loss from whooping cough and it was noted that both height and weight were on the 50th centile for age so a referral to the surgeons was arranged. There are three reasons for a testis not being sited in the scrotum (Table 15.6).

Table 15.6
Classification of undescended testis

Retractile (normal)
A normal testis drawn up towards the external ring by a strong cremasteric reflex
Etopic
A testis in the wrong place after a normal descent through the inguinal canal and the external ring (e.g. the superficial inguinal pouch)
Maldescended
A testis which has incompletely descended (e.g. intra-abdominal or lying in the inguinal canal

The surgical registrar found a hypoplastic scrotum on the left, and was initially unable to feel the left testis. However, he was just able to coax the testis down to the end of the inguinal canal and feel it at the external ring— by drawing his left fingers down the line of the inguinal canal. The testis came nowhere near the scrotum (excluding a retractile testis), and since it had not emerged from the external ring he concluded it was maldescended— rather like a hand caught in a sleeve.

Comment

The long-term hazards of maldescended testes are trauma, malignant change and torsion. If the condition is bilateral (20 per cent) there is a risk of infertility. Since no change in position will occur after 9 months of age, Justin had an orchidopexy a few months later. There is a risk of thermal damage or trauma, so all undescended testes should be treated before 5 years of age (1–3 years is optimal). At operation the testicular vessels and vasa deferentia are mobilized and the testes placed in the scrotum.

The aim of surgery is to enhance fertility, as nearly all adults with bilateral undescended testes are infertile even though they have normal sex hormone production. Fertility rates are assessed on results of operations carried out 20 years ago when such children were treated at a later age. They suggest a 40 per cent chance of being fertile in adult life when there are bilaterally undescended testes.